Quality Caring
in Nursing

D1516143

DATE DUE

GAYLORD   PRINTED IN U.S.A.

Joanne R. Duffy, PhD, RN, FAAN, has over 35 years of nursing experience encompassing clinical, administrative, and academic roles. She is currently a Professor at the Indiana University School of Nursing in Indianapolis, IN, and a Fellow in the American Academy of Nursing.

Dr. Duffy has coordinated three graduate nursing programs (critical care, care management, and nursing administration) and was a former Division Director of a school of nursing. She has held various administrative positions directing critical care and transplantation nursing services as well as being the founding director of a nurse-run Center for Outcomes Analysis. She has published extensively across nursing literature, but is best known for her work in maximizing patient outcomes. Dr. Duffy was the first to link nurse caring to patient outcomes and has designed the Caring Assessment Tool in multiple versions. She is a recipient of several nursing awards, a frequent guest speaker, and a Magnet Appraiser.

Dr. Duffy was the Principal Investigator on the national demonstration project, Relationship-Centered Caring in Acute Care, where the Quality-Caring Model© is being evaluated at two sites in terms of patient, nurse, and system outcomes. She provided direction for the Telehomecare and Heart Failure Outcomes project. She was a consultant to the American Nurses Association (ANA) in the development and implementation of the National Database of Nursing Quality Indicators (NDNQI) and is currently the chair of the National League for Nursing's (NLN) Nursing Educational Research Advisory Council.

Quality Caring in Nursing

Applying Theory to Clinical Practice, Education, and Leadership

JOANNE R. DUFFY, PhD, RN, FAAN

Stoxen Library Dickinson State Univ.

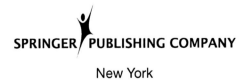

SPRINGER PUBLISHING COMPANY

New York

Copyright © 2009 Springer Publishing Company, LLC

All rights reserved.

No part of this publication may be reproduced, stored in a retrieval system, or transmitted in any form or by any means, electronic, mechanical, photocopying, recording, or otherwise, without the prior permission of the publisher or authorization through payment of the appropriate fees to the Copyright Clearance Center, Inc., 222 Rosewood Drive, Danvers, MA 01923, 978-750-8400, fax 978-646-8600, info@copyright.com or on the web at www.copyright.com.

Springer Publishing Company, LLC
11 West 42nd Street
New York, NY 10036
www.springerpub.com

Acquisitions Editor: Allan Graubard
Production Editor: Julia Rosen
Cover design: Steve Pisano
Composition: Apex CoVantage, LLC

Ebook ISBN: 978-0-8261-2129-5

08 09 10 11/ 5 4 3 2 1

Library of Congress Cataloging-in-Publication Data

Duffy, Joanne R.
  Quality caring in nursing : applying theory to clinical practice, education, and leadership / Joanne R. Duffy.
    p. ; cm.
  Includes bibliographical references and index.
  ISBN 978-0-8261-2128-8 (alk. paper)
  1. Nursing—Standards.   2. Clinical competence.   I. Title.
  [DNLM: 1. Nursing Care—standards.   2. Nursing Theory.   3. Quality Assurance, Health Care—standards.   WY 100 D867q 2009]
  RT85.5.D82   2009
  610.73—dc22   2008038974

Printed in Canada by Transcontinental

The author and the publisher of this Work have made every effort to use sources believed to be reliable to provide information that is accurate and compatible with the standards generally accepted at the time of publication. Because medical science is continually advancing, our knowledge base continues to expand. Therefore, as new information becomes available, changes in procedures become necessary. We recommend that the reader always consult current research and specific institutional policies before performing any clinical procedure. The author and publisher shall not be liable for any special, consequential, or exemplary damages resulting, in whole or in part, from the readers' use of, or reliance on, the information contained in this book. The publisher has no responsibility for the persistence or accuracy of URLs for external or third-party Internet Web sites referred to in this publication and does not guarantee that any content on such Web sites is, or will remain, accurate or appropriate.

Contents

Foreword

Joanne Duffy's work in theory-guided caring and issues of quality caring, in education, practice, and research, spans more than two decades of scholarship and sustained focus. Her scholarship in this area has deepened and expanded with each turn of her career, culminating in this comprehensive book, which demonstrates her unique contributions to this field of increasing importance. Her book offers a coherent, theoretical, and research-guided framework for quality nursing caring in practice, education, and leadership; a foundational, timeless, yet transformative framework of substance related to caring and quality, for which systems and society yearn at this point in the history of nursing and health care.

Here, Duffy's classic model, Quality Caring and Quality Nursing Practice (The Quality-Caring Model©), is revisited and reconsidered. It is grounded in a comprehensive framework that addresses and encompasses caring for self, patients, families, each other, and communities. The power of relationships, the teaching and learning of caring, and caring leadership are addressed in such a way that the reader is invited both into conceptual and theoretical ideas along with an opportunity to engage in specific skills of evaluating and researching caring. In this way, the book offers the most contemporary literature on caring as well as action steps for informed engagement by students and scholars alike.

Duffy's book brings coherence and congruence between and among professional values, knowledge, and behaviors of caring in nursing and health care generally. In the end, Duffy's "quality caring" brings new meaning to *quality* and to *caring*. At the same time, the book is both power-filled in its focus as well as empowering. Any reader of the work is invited into an open space that reconnects the heart of nursing with the heart of caring science scholarship. As a significant and timely contribution to nursing and caring science, Duffy incorporates into the book a new level of values, philosophical and ethical orientations, along with knowledge and understanding if not wisdom. Indeed, Joanne Duffy's work and life career in this area continue to advance and elevate nursing and quality caring to a new place in the maturity of nursing as both a discipline and profession.

Jean Watson, PhD, RN, AHN-BC, FAAN
Distinguished Professor of Nursing
Murchinson-Scoville Endowed Chair in Caring Science
University of Colorado, Denver
College of Nursing
and
Founder/Director
Watson Caring Science Institute
Boulder, Colorado
www.uchsc.edu/nursing/caring
www.watsoncaringscience.org
jean.watson@uchsc.edu

Preface

Patients and families are suffering today not only from their illnesses but from the health care system itself. Fragmented processes, medical errors, and lack of caring relationships with their health care providers create uncertainty, unnecessary stress, discomfort, functional decline, dissatisfaction with care, and unnecessary financial burdens. Evidence of this can be found in conversations in hospital waiting rooms, newspaper articles, consumer magazines, and professional journals. Dedicated time spent with patients and families at the bedside, in medical offices, at nursing homes, or schools is limited and often rushed and impersonal. Patients and families, at some of the most vulnerable times of life, are frequently left to wonder if they are safe and who will be there for them when they need it most. The foundational caring value of health professionals has been marginalized as modern health care, with its emphasis on diagnostic testing, medications, and procedures, has shifted its attention to tasks, technology, and costs.

This incongruity between the professional values and behaviors of health care professionals is serious and may be linked to poor health care outcomes. Not only has the reduced time spent "in relationship" challenged patients and families but health care providers themselves, particularly professional nurses, who may be jeopardizing their professional integrity (acting in accordance with the core values of one's profession, such as the value of caring in nursing) leading to dissatisfaction and lack of motivation surrounding work. This is particularly difficult for the new graduate nurse who has been educated "to care" and then finds himself/herself working in a department that is rushed, has little supportive infrastructure, is focused on throughput and staffing, and offers few incentives for professional development.

Nurses, who are the largest group of health care providers and are with patients and families for the longest periods, are in a unique position to advance a more relationship-oriented health care system. Through theory-based practice models, values-based curricula, and relationship-centered leadership (including redesigned patient care delivery systems and governance models focused on the primacy of relationships), the gap between professional values and professional practice can be narrowed. Never has it been more important to advance this agenda, for nursing itself may be in jeopardy.

This book provides an overview of the quality crisis in health care, a theoretical foundation for action, and application at several levels. The intent of the book is to raise awareness of nursing's significance in improving the quality of the health care system. Additionally, it is a call to professional nurses, *all nurses,* to action. Safe, quality health care and meaningful work are at stake.

Through exploration of theoretical concepts drawn from multiple sources, a model is revealed that has the capacity to honor nursing's most deeply held value: caring. The important relationships with self, community, patients and families, and the health care team are illuminated and redefined for current practice. Applying the model in practice, education, and leadership offers possibilities for caring-healing-protective environments where genuine professional nursing can flourish. Using the model as a foundation for research may point to new evidence of nursing's contribution to quality health care.

Part 1 focuses on nursing's unique contribution to health care and highlights the value of nursing to the current quality crisis. It reviews the original Quality-Caring Model©, a postmodern middle range theory of caring. Part 2 concentrates on those relationships necessary for quality caring. Relationships with self, patients and families, members of the health care team, and the community are described using great detail and examples. Part 3 centers on the application of quality caring in clinical practice, nursing education, research, and leadership. Finally, the future of nursing and health care is forecasted as complex, interactive, and integrative. Using this background, the Quality-Caring Model© is revised.

HOW TO USE THIS BOOK

The text is intended for use by nursing students, particularly graduate students, and nursing scholars as well as clinical nurses, nurse educators, nurse researchers, and those in nursing leadership positions. Each chapter contains an introductory section followed by specific narratives holding new information or applications. Areas of special emphasis are boxed to highlight their importance while specific Calls to Action are included at the end of each chapter. The text offers multiple case examples and includes reflective questions and applications for use in formal education programs, continuing education, workshops and conferences, and general clinical practice. Although these additions are organized for students, educators, and nurse leaders, they are not mutually exclusive and may be used by nurses in many different roles. The Appendices provide additional resources for those interested in caring clinical practice, education, and leadership.

The text begins with disturbing facts about quality and the state of professional nursing practice particularly in hospitals; yet, the value of professional nursing to quality health care and society is repeatedly emphasized. Using this period of disillusionment in health care as an opportunity for growth, professional nurses at all levels are called to remember and renew their commitment to caring relationships as the cornerstone of their practice.

Acknowledgments

To the five men in my life . . . my husband, Steve, who embodies caring and has lovingly cared for me during our long marriage; my son, Kevin, who values history and the arts and who uses humor to lighten my world; and my three baby grandsons—Matthew, Brian, and Jake—who delight me with their smiles and hugs. And to my two daughters . . . Erin, who now shares the wonder of motherhood with me; and Meghan, who appreciates the French heritage of her grandmother, my mother, who is with God, watching over us all.

Nursing's Unique Contribution to Health Care

1 Quality and Nursing Practice

Quality in a product or service is not what the provider puts in. It is what the customer gets out.

—Peter F. Drucker

Keywords: quality, health care, nursing

THE CRISIS OF QUALITY IN HEALTH CARE

In the now famous Institute of Medicine (IOM) reports, health care quality and safety threats were widely acknowledged (IOM, 1999, 2001). In fact, it was estimated that almost 100,000 Americans die annually in hospitals due to errors. In another report, it was recognized that 18% of hospitalized patients experience a serious medication error (Davis et al., 2004). Furthermore, using the Centers for Disease Control (CDC) reported health care–associated infections, an estimated 1.7 million infections and 99,000 associated deaths occur each year (Klevens et al., 2007). A landmark RAND corporation study completed in 2006 reported that Americans only receive half of recommended medical care and that having health insurance was not a ticket to quality care (Asch et al., 2006). Reports of Americans choosing hospitals in other countries are rising (Corchado & Iliff, 2007), and in one northeastern state, a teaching

3

hospital was fined for operating on the wrong side of patients' heads *for the third time* (Associated Press, 2007b). A surprise Joint Commission check at another prominent northeastern hospital found numerous problems with medication safety and inconsistent handwashing (Kowalczyk, 2007). And, in long-term care, "serious problems concerning quality of care . . . continue to affect residents of this country's nursing homes" (IOM, 2001, p. 2). On November 29, 2007, the U.S. federal government publicly listed 54 nursing homes as the worst in their states in order to stimulate improvement in their services (Associated Press, 2007a).

Needless pain, disability, anxiety, and additional costs attributed to poor-quality health care threaten Americans as they age, attempt to manage chronic illness, and deal with issues such as violence, obesity, and substance abuse. What is even worse is that several years after these reports highlighted the rising health care quality crisis, many Americans say they do not believe the nation's health care has improved; in fact, 40% believe it has gotten worse (Clancy, Farquhar, & Sharp, 2005).

Since 2001, quality improvement initiatives and research have documented that while many indicators of quality are improving, many more remain problematic. For example, in a recent supplement to the *Joint Commission Journal of Quality and Patient Safety* (Institute for Healthcare Improvement, 2007), authors cited fatigue, inadequate nurse staffing levels, and emergency department crowding as persistent threats to patient safety, and the 2007 *Health Grades Hospital Study* reported that "significant variation in the quality of care provided by the nation's hospitals has persisted over the last eight years despite numerous quality initiatives at the hospital, local, state and federal levels" (p. 4). For example, among the 18 conditions studied during the prior year, 266,604 potentially preventable deaths occurred among Medicare recipients (Health Grades, Inc., 2007). Additionally, hospitals located in the East North Central region (Illinois, Indiana, Michigan, Ohio, and Wisconsin) had the best performance, while hospitals located in the East South Central (Alabama, Kentucky, Missouri, and Tennessee) had the worst performance with respect to risk-adjusted mortality. And in the Joint Commission on Accreditation of Healthcare Organizations' (JCAHO) annual report, although measurable improvement in quality and safety was noted, much room for improvement remained (JCAHO, 2007). In this report, consistent performance in several quality measures was less than expected, and continued variability in performance of hospitals by state was noted. In long-term care, the problem is much worse. In a government report of nursing home inspections, more than

22% actually caused harm to their residents (General Accounting Office, 2003).

Although the Agency for Healthcare Research and Quality (AHRQ), the JCAHO, the Institute for Healthcare Improvement (IHI), and the National Quality Forum (NQF) are making great strides through funding research and setting quality standards, the value of the American health care system has declined. It suffers from an older industrialized model, lack of communication and coordination, major safety concerns, inconsistent follow-up, insufficient numbers and education of workers, poor reimbursement systems, and lack of concern for the individual being treated. Most disturbing is this last component. In a recent account of his hospitalization, a national radio talk show host said, "the nurse didn't help, he just stood there and drummed his fingers against the door, made no eye contact, and walked in front of me." And when the same patient expressed his fear about his inability to breathe, another nurse replied, "you look like you're breathing fine to me" (Beck, 2008). The radio host went on to describe his fear of the night, the constant messages that he didn't matter, and his loss of dignity as his wife was forced to clean him in a dirty shower stall. While admitting that he was taking several pain killers, the radio host called this lack of patient-centeredness a "compassion pandemic" and went on to say that he experienced the health care system at its very worse.

Health care today is rushed, impersonal, and often stress-provoking. For example, it is still the norm to see a health care provider in a busy office/clinic for a few minutes at best and leave without questions answered, adequate knowledge, lack of understanding in self-care, or prevention of future illness. Hospital emergency department overcrowding and long delays are common (Trzeciak & Rivers, 2003), and access to inpatient beds often requires multiple phone calls and often painfully long waits in hallways. Sick persons are expected to obey the rules set by hospital staff; for example, the timing of procedures. A male patient recovering from thoracic surgery recently relayed that he was awakened at 3:15 A.M. on his second postoperative night for a chest X-ray because "we had time to do it." Communications and handoffs between hospital departments and nursing shifts are often inaccurate or untimely resulting in missed or lost information, many times influencing errors (Hughes & Clancy, 2007). The individualized human concern and relationship context one would expect from health care professionals is frequently forgotten in the busyness of modern health care systems. Furthermore, mutual decision making about the care received or alternatives to suggested care are almost nonexistent. In the business world, such lack of attention to customer expectations and needs would most certainly lead to bankruptcy and eventual collapse!

So, despite the most costly health care system in the world, the U.S. health care enterprise underperforms and, some would say, even causes harm to patients and families. The reality is that American health care professionals remain in denial about the quality of care they provide and the somewhat overt problems that plague the system. The education of physicians and nurses, while slowly changing, remains fact-based and rule-dominated; providers themselves are overworked and do not regularly practice their own self-caring; hospitals and long-term care facilities are slow to change; and reimbursement pressures plague the system.

QUALITY AND PROFESSIONAL NURSING PRACTICE

As the largest group of health care professionals, nurses contribute in positive and negative ways to the health care quality problem. Nurses have intimate knowledge of patient needs, and the continuous interactions nurses maintain with patients and families uniquely position them to positively influence their hospital experiences and resultant outcomes. In fact, the IHI's *Transforming Care at the Bedside* initiative supports that "RNs play a central role in ensuring the quality of hospital care" (Rutherford, Lee, & Greiner, 2004, p. 2). While few reports were found in the professional literature regarding poor nurse quality, perceptions of a decline in quality among hospital nurses and patients have risen in recent years.

In 2001, the Milbank Memorial Fund published a report by Dr. Claire Fagin of the University of Pennsylvania to document these perceptions. The report synthesized research studies, newspaper and magazine articles, and personal experience to conclude that "there is considerable evidence that nurses and families are very concerned about the erosion of care and fearful about hospital safety" (Fagin, 2001, p. 3). One aspect of the report suggested that the reduction in the amount of time professional nurses spend in direct patient care was a cause. The growing use of unlicensed assistive personnel (UAP) since the mid-90s has contributed to this perception. Coupled with the nursing shortage (Beurhaus, Donelan, Ulrich, Norman, & Dittus, 2005), the perception persists that professional nurses are less involved with direct care and more often observed administering medications or supervising others in direct care (Duffy, Baldwin, & Mastorovich, 2007). Personal experience by this author and others substantiates that hospital professional nurses have little time to spend listening to patients' concerns, coming to know them as unique human beings, educating them about their illnesses, and attending to their needs for comfort, support, and security. In fact, some health care providers advise taking another health professional or reliable family member to the hospital during admissions *to ensure high-quality care* (Consumer Reports, 2003; Trafford, 2001).

A doctorally prepared nurse speaking at a national conference recently recounted her experience with her mother who was admitted to an acute care hospital for a surgical procedure (Amendolair, 2008). The mother was limited in her hearing, and the nurses, who used a computer to document assessment data, faced the computer rather than the patient each time they inquired about her last bowel movement. The patient could not hear them so she didn't respond, and the nurses did not validate the patient's answer, so they charted seven times over the course of three days that she had a bowel movement when, in fact, she had not. Eventually, the patient became impacted.

Another nurse wrote of her experiences receiving nursing care after major surgery for uterine cancer in a major teaching hospital. "From admission through discharge, I was appalled with the lack of knowledgeable and compassionate care . . . unfortunately, I had to provide the knowledge component for my own care. For example, I diagnosed my paralytic ileus, since not one nurse placed a stethoscope on my belly to assess for bowel sounds after major abdominal surgery, and I kept track of my own intake and output and determined when I was dehydrated" (Todaro-Franceschi, 2007, p. 230). She went on to say it took her a long time to heal, and she was saddened by the state of nursing she experienced.

In one grounded theory approach to better understanding patients' experiences of "not so good" nursing care, the author found that care delivered routinely, that was unrelated to patient needs and performed in an impersonal manner, was considered by patients to be of lower quality (Attree, 2001). Using a convenient sample of 80 patients and 30 nurses in acute care, a descriptive study in Sweden found that "RNs had considerable difficulty identifying the needs of their patients," and emotions/spirituality and nutrition had the lowest ratings (Florin, Ehrenberg, & Ehnfors, 2005, p. 9). In another Swedish descriptive study, patients reported care quality in the emergency department as fairly good with several areas needing improvement (Muntlin, Gunningberg, & Carlsson, 2006).

An important U.S. study of the quality of nursing care found significant variations in nursing care quality (Chang et al., 2002). Using a retrospective medical records peer review process, 291 heart failure (HF) and 283 stroke patients' records were randomly selected from 5 states. Trained nurse peer-reviewers used a quality rating scale based on the nursing process to evaluate the overall quality of nursing care. Findings revealed that systematic variations in nursing care were linked to hospital type (smaller hospitals provided significantly worse nursing care) and geography (more rural locations were associated with worse nursing care); furthermore, variations in care were more pronounced in HF patients than those patients with strokes. Although the sample of records is from the 1980s, this study is important because it documents nursing variation in care for the first time and demonstrates the inconsistent application of the nursing process. With the current approach to assigning some clinical responsibilities to unlicensed assistive personnel, the nursing shortage, and higher acuity in American hospitals, one would suspect that these problems persist and may even be worse.

Kalisch (2006) used a qualitative approach to determine whether opportunities for nursing care were regularly overlooked and the reasons for such missed care on American hospital medical-surgical units. Using two hospitals and focus group interviews with nurses and nursing assistants, Kalisch found nine areas of regularly missed nursing care. They were: ambulation, turning, feeding, patient teaching, discharge planning, emotional support, hygiene, intake and output documentation, and surveillance. Although limited by the sample, this study's results are profound in that the reasons for missed care were often related to the nurses themselves. For example, ineffective delegation, "it's not my job syndrome," habit, the amount of time involved, and denial were cited as some reasons for missed care. Furthermore, these areas of omitted nursing care may have untoward effects on patient outcomes. This study's results point out that, in this sample, behaviors traditionally associated with good nursing care were often overlooked or not completed and that nurses failed to follow up on delegated tasks and used denial as a coping mechanism to deal with missed care.

In another qualitative study in Iceland, subjects who experienced nurses who provided bad quality care described the nurses as indifferent, having no initiative, or having a negative attitude (Thorsteinsson, 2002). Those subjects also described poor quality nursing care as producing negative effects such as anger or stress. Newspaper accounts of poor quality nursing care in hospitals and nursing homes are abundant, and many have been attributed primarily to the recent nursing shortage. However, experiences with noncaring nurses have been documented for a long time. As early as 1986, noncaring behaviors by nurses were cited in the professional literature (Reiman, 1986). In this report, Reiman described a nurse's interaction with a 21-year-old woman with lupus erythematosus as discouraging. She went on to say, "it is frightening to realize that at a time when patients are so vulnerable, nurses are perceived as doing those very things that make patients even more vulnerable" (p. 33). Kelly (1988) reported that noncaring behaviors by hospital nurses existed and accounted for needless patient and family anxiety. The descriptions of nursing behaviors as rough, causing unnecessary pain, and void of concern resulted in loss of human dignity for the patients in this sample. Lastly, Proudfoot (1983) spoke to nurses as having "hurry sickness."

One would have to ask, "Has anything changed?" Despite almost three decades of study of the essential caring behaviors required for expert nursing practice (Benner & Wrubel, 1989; Boykin & Schoenhofer, 1993; Leininger, 1998; Roach, 1984; Swanson, 1991; Watson, 1979, 1985), caring practices by professional nurses remain problematic. They are present but hidden in daily practice by some nurses, kept separated from the "doing" aspect of nursing, and seemingly absent in others. Along with the decrease in numbers of professional nurses and the rushed, task-oriented, impersonal nature of health care, it seems as if caring in nursing has been devalued. In reality, the very foundation of the profession may be broken (see Figure 1.1).

So, while solid evidence about inadequate nursing care is limited, perceptions exist among nurses, physicians, and patients and families about the declining professional nurse role particularly in hospitals. Quantitative evidence from which to judge the nature of nursing quality or its relationship to patient outcomes has been scarce.

INDICATORS OF NURSING QUALITY

Indicators, or measures, that specifically reflect nursing care are considered nursing-sensitive and are used to evaluate and demonstrate to the public how nursing contributes to the quality and safety of health care recipients, particularly those who are hospitalized. Dr. Norma Lang pioneered the quality assurance effort in nursing beginning in the early 1970s, developing a model of nursing quality assessment, publishing in peer-reviewed journals, and conducting numerous workshops advocating

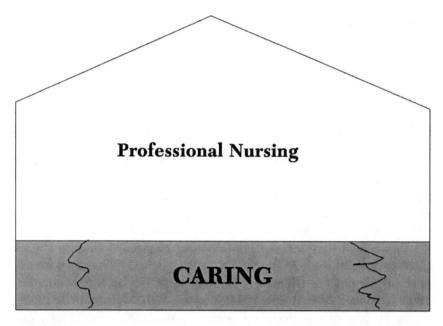

Numbers &   Practice environment
Credentials of RNs   Task focus

Figure 1.1 Nursing's fractured foundation.

for a standardized nursing language and consulting in both nursing education and nursing service (Lang, 2003). She helped enhance the knowledge of evidence-based nursing and provided a lens from which to view and improve nursing quality.

In 1995, the American Nurses Association (ANA) embarked on a study of nursing-sensitive indicators from which they could track data linked to nursing care. Using a series of focus groups and a Delphi approach, the ANA identified 10 indicators for acute care while an additional 10 indicators for community-based nursing were added in 2000 (Gallagher, 2005; Gallagher & Rowell, 2003). (See Tables 1.1 and 1.2 for a list of the ANA indicators.)

The ANA's investment in the program *Patient Safety Nurse Quality,* a national comparative database of nursing-sensitive quality indicators intended to measure the impact of professional nurses on health care outcomes, is used by hospitals to improve the quality of their nursing services. The database, known as the National Database of Nursing Quality Indicators (NDNQI), uses the structure, process, and outcomes indicators that reflect nursing's contribution to patient care (ANA, 2000;

Table 1.1

AMERICAN NURSES ASSOCIATION'S ACUTE CARE NURSING-SENSITIVE INDICATORS

Nursing hours

Nosocomial infections

Nurse satisfaction

Patient injuries (falls)

Pressure ulcers

Staff mix

Patient satisfaction (overall)

Patient satisfaction (education)

Patient satisfaction (nursing care)

Patient satisfaction (pain management)

From "Claiming the Future of Nursing Through Nursing-Sensitive Quality Indicators," by R. M. Gallagher and P. Rowell, 2003, *Nursing Administration Quarterly, 27*(4), 273–284.

Table 1.2

COMMUNITY-BASED, NONACUTE CARE INDICATORS

Pain management

Consistency of communication

Staff mix (use of services)

Client satisfaction

Prevention of tobacco use (risk reduction)

Cardiovascular prevention (risk reduction)

Caregiver activity (protective factors)

Identification of primary caregiver (protective factors)

ADL/IADL (level of function)

Psychosocial interaction (level of function)

From "Claiming the Future of Nursing Through Nursing-Sensitive Quality Indicators," by R. M. Gallagher and P. Rowell, 2003, *Nursing Administration Quarterly, 27*(4), 273–284.

Donabedian, 1966). This initiative has led to the *Nursing Care Report Card for Acute Care* with standardized data submission forms and routine reporting (ANA, 1995). More than 1,200 U.S. hospitals participate in the project, now housed within the ANA's National Center for Nursing Quality, and annual conferences are held to assist users and showcase the latest research.

In 2004, the NQF published a landmark report documenting a set of 15 nursing-sensitive performance measures endorsed through consensus. The voluntary standards were intended to be used by providers to identify opportunities for improvement so that consumers and purchasers of care could assess the quality of nursing care in hospitals (NQF, 2004). (See Table 1.3 for the complete list of performance standards.)

In a review of these standards three years later, the NQF found that several of the standards are in use, but because of some of the challenges they pose in collection and reporting, the extent to which they are used is not clear. Although the sample size was small and the results not generalizable, findings from this NQF report revealed 50% of the respondents adopted 7 (or half of the standards), while only 13 of 31 (or 42%) collected all 15 (Kurtzman & Corrigan, 2007). One recommendation from these results that purports to reflect nursing's impact on high-quality care through public reporting and incentive systems has led to a revision of Medicare reimbursement for patients with hospital-acquired adverse outcomes. Beginning in October 2008, Medicare will eliminate additional payments for several inpatient conditions that are traditionally associated with high-quality nursing care (Robert Wood Johnson Foundation, 2007). This ruling promises to affect hospital organizational priorities and the work lives of professional nurses. It will also showcase indicators of nursing quality that for the first time will be tied to reimbursement and may be publicly available.

Nursing research and the measurement of nursing quality in acute and nonacute settings have increased considerably over the last few years. For example, evidence now exists linking nurse staffing and selected quality indicators (Aiken, Clarke, & Sloane, 2002a, 2002b; Aiken, Sochalski, & Lake, 1997; Dunton, Grajewski, Taunton, & Moore, 2004; Needleman & Buerhaus, 2003; Needleman, Buerhaus, Mattke, Stewart, & Zelevinsky, 2002), the educational level of hospital nurses and selected patient outcomes (Aiken, Clarke, Cheung, Sloane, & Silber, 2003), the nurse work environment and patients' satisfaction with their nursing care (Vahey, Aiken, Sloane, Clarke, & Vargas, 2004), nurse staffing and the quality of nursing care in hospitals (Sochalski, 2004), and the working

Table 1.3

NATIONAL QUALITY FORUM'S VOLUNTARY CONSENSUS STANDARDS FOR NURSING-SENSITIVE CARE

1. Death among surgical in-patients with treatable serious complications (failure to rescue)
2. Pressure ulcer prevalence
3. Falls prevalence
4. Falls with injury
5. Restraint prevalence (vest and limb only)
6. Urinary catheter–associated urinary tract infection for intensive care unit (ICU) patients
7. Central line catheter–associated bloodstream infection rate for ICU and high-risk nursery (HRN) patients
8. Ventilator-associated pneumonia for ICU and HRN patients
9. Smoking cessation counseling for acute myocardial infarction
10. Smoking cessation counseling for heart failure
11. Smoking cessation counseling for pneumonia
12. Skill mix (RN, LVN/LPN, UAP, and contract)
13. Nursing care hours per patient day (RN, LPN, and UAP)
14. Practice Environment Scale–Nursing Work Index (composite and five subscales)
15. Voluntary turnover

From *National Voluntary Consensus Standards for Nursing-Sensitive Care: An Initial Performance Measure Set. A Consensus Report,* by the National Quality Forum, 2004, Washington, DC: National Quality Forum.

hours of nurses and patient safety (Rogers, Hwang, Scott, Aiken, & Dinges, 2004). In the nonacute environment, evidence points to specialized advance practice interventions and improved patient outcomes and health care costs (Brooten, Brooks, Madigan, & Youngblut, 1998; Brooten et al., 2001; Brooten, Youngblut, Deatrick, Naylor, & York, 2003; Brooten, Youngblut, Kutcher, & Bobo, 2004; Naylor et al., 1999). While this research is significant, much more needs to be done to demonstrate nursing's link to quality health care, including more widespread dissemination (Naylor, 2003).

From the patient's point of view, quality nursing care is primarily process-oriented, most notably "being with." In their study of 1,470 acute care patients, Lynn, McMillen, and Sidana (2007) found that technical competence was assumed and the process aspects of care were most often cited as indicators of nurse quality. However, current evidence shows that registered nurses (RNs) spend less than half their work time in direct patient care at a time when patients are living longer with cyclical chronic diseases and are expected to engage in self-care (Duffy, 2005; Hendrickson, Doddato, & Kovner, 1990; Linden & English, 1994; Urden & Roode, 1997). While staffing may be a factor in nursing quality, other factors such as motivation, leadership, educational preparation, the work environment, or culture may also contribute to nursing quality. The focus on task-completion, documentation, and technical competence has curbed the processes of nursing, such as mutual problem-solving, encouragement, continuous monitoring, ongoing evaluation, teaching-learning, coordination, and intervening in a compassionate manner.

THE VALUE OF PROFESSIONAL NURSING PRACTICE

The word *value* connotes worth, and as such, the question being asked today is, "in an economically constrained system, what is the significance of professional nursing?" After all, other professionals are often seen providing aspects of health care such as respiratory care, physical therapy, occupational therapy, and social work services. Patient care technicians have been trained to provide hygienic care and even ambulate postoperative patients. When posed the question in a recent graduate class of practicing RNs, the answer was "we spend the shift passing meds" (personal communication, The Catholic University of America, 2006). When reminded that medication techs could be trained in that behavior, the RNs in the class were astounded! On the face of it, it appeared as if professional nursing was almost nonexistent in acute care. In some cases, it is.

The reality today is that nursing is in crisis. Not only is the profession suffering from a worker shortage, some would say it has lost its soul (Duffy & Hoskins, 2003). As more and more of its traditional

(continued)

activities have been progressively given away to other health professionals and increasing reliance on tasks has emerged, nursing seems to lack a unique function. The very essence of nursing (caring) (Watson, 1979, 1985) is not routinely honored in the day-to-day activities of professional nurses. Yet, nursing remains the primary reason patients come to hospitals; their roles in assessing and continuous monitoring, clinical decision making, providing comfort, educating patients and families about their illness, and maintaining a safe and therapeutic environment are paramount.

Aiken (2005b) states that the two most important functions of nurses, that of surveillance for early detection of adverse events, complications, and medical errors as well as mobilizing institutional resources for timely intervention and rescue, are keys to safe and quality health care outcomes. Furthermore, professional nurses are often the "coordinators" of services between multiple members of the health care team. In this function, nurses collaborate with others and often negotiate difficult relationships. Yet, sadly, professional nurses are often observed doing countless tasks such as administering medications, supervising others, and documenting. And while these are certainly aspects of the role, the unique characteristics of initiating, cultivating, and sustaining caring relationships with patients and families as a foundation for clinical decision making are oftentimes lacking (Duffy & Hoskins, 2003).

A public opinion survey sponsored by the Robert Wood Johnson Foundation (RWJF; 2006) found that "Americans consider nursing a vital component of quality health care" (p. 1). Recent research has renewed the interest in professional nursing as an important contributor to safe and quality care. More specifically, the risks of death and failure to rescue patients from complications increase by 7% every time one patient is added to a hospital nurse's workload (RWJF, 2006). Additionally, a 10% increase in a hospital's proportion of nurses with bachelor's degrees decreases mortality and failure to rescue by 5% (RWJF, 2006). These data provide important quantitative evidence of the value of professional nursing and ensure that nursing remains on the national health care agenda (Aiken, 2005a). While the numbers and educational credentials of nurses seem to be linked to important health outcomes, understanding how the processes of nursing or specific nursing actions influence patient outcomes will enhance the knowledge base regarding the value of professional nursing care.

Preliminary research has indicated positive relationships between caring nurse–patient relationships and specific patient outcomes (Burt, 2007; Duffy, 1992; Latham, 1996; Swan, 1998; Wolf, Colahan, & Costello, 1998; Yeakel, Maljanian, Bohannon, & Coulombe, 2003). Although these studies are limited by sample size and methodology, there is a growing group of hospital and nursing administrators who have adopted caring professional practice models as the foundation for nursing practice (Dingman, Williams, Fosbinder, & Warnnick, 1999; Duffy, Baldwin, & Mastorowich, 2007; Watson, 2006). These models emphasize nursing's primary role as relationship-building and provide the infrastructure to facilitate the authentic work of nursing. Patient, nurse, and system outcomes in institutions using a nurse caring model will demonstrate nursing's unique value to the health care system.

OPPORTUNITIES FOR ENHANCING THE QUALITY OF NURSING PRACTICE

The increasing evidence that nursing is a worthy contributor to safe and quality health care is long overdue. While nurses have always known that they are the frontline advocates for high quality and safe care, evidence supporting this link was weak. Continued, methodologically strong research is crucial for enhancing the quality of nursing practice. For example, testing theory-based professional practice models and nursing interventions focused on patient safety and quality in various patient populations is urgently needed to showcase the efforts of professional nursing. Dedicated nursing research teams with expertise in differing populations who are committed to safety and quality questions working efficiently could expedite such studies. Participatory action research and demonstration projects involving practicing staff nurses using academic/service partnerships may facilitate more creative solutions that can be implemented and evaluated sooner.

Strengthening the nursing workforce through education by providing meaningful experiential opportunities that enable practicing staff nurses to complete baccalaureate degrees efficiently will add to the proportion of more educated nurses. Certification credentials and continuing education in information technology and research skills will enable RNs to capitalize on existing evidence. Although presently underfunded, more nursing educational research will be needed to build a portfolio demonstrating how nurses learn best and what personal characteristics of nurses most impact safe and quality health care (National League for Nursing, 2007).

Migrating away from fact-based learning to values-based learning will help nursing students examine their own values and those of their chosen profession. Caring, as the most often described value associated with nursing, must remain a major thrust of nursing education. A strong liberal arts foundation combined with caring competencies and experiential learning methods will strengthen tomorrow's professional nurses. Frequent opportunities for critical reflection (both individual and group) will enhance self-awareness and contribute to more caring practice (Bulman & Schutz, 2004). Strong student–faculty relationships of a caring nature will demonstrate to students the essential core value of nursing. Using caring student–faculty relationships as the core of learning may decrease student anxiety and create more cohesive learning (Pullen, Murray, & McGee, 2001; Schaffer & Juarez, 1996). This includes caring in Web-enhanced environments. While the use of technology offers opportunities for efficiency (Simpson, 2008), it can best do so when applied within a caring framework. Finally, educational program evaluation including student caring competencies will better inform faculty how to revise curricula to meet the caring learning needs of students (Duffy, 2005).

Nurses holding leadership positions (at all levels) must ask themselves on a daily basis if they are staffing for safe and quality care. Routine involvement in overseeing the quality of nursing care, including making assignments based on competency for specific clinical situations, rounding, and actively seeking to improve nursing care, must become the primary focus of nurse leaders. Within this primary focus of continuously seeking to improve quality, nursing leaders must value nurse caring by ensuring that the majority of nursing time is spent in direct care activities. According to Aiken (2005b), "good nurse–patient relationships are at the heart of safe and effective hospital care" (p. 186). Redesigning the work environment to provide more time for direct RN–patient interaction is vital. According to the Institute for Healthcare Improvement's *Transforming Care at the Bedside*, a goal of clinicians is to spend 70% of time in direct patient care (Rutherford, Lee, & Greiner, 2007). Such redesign requires rethinking the work content of RNs so that patient needs are primary. Enhancing the work environment to include focused reminders for centering, creating places for reflection and regrouping, and innovative opportunities for on-the-spot problem resolution will boost nurses' autonomy and position them to more effectively influence decisions. Finally, stimulating career development activities that incentivize caring praxis are long overdue.

At the practice level, nursing is at a crossroads in its professional evolution. In one respect, it has become devalued and relegated to task-oriented service. On the other hand, professional nursing is on the brink of reclaiming caring as the basis of practice, questioning how care is delivered, and assuring that nursing care is grounded in scientific evidence. It is within this realm of nursing that its future can be secured and its recipients honored. The relational aspect of nursing is highly valued by patients and families; it must receive equal if not more priority in the workplace (Bikker & Thompson, 2006). With the patient and family at the core, nurses who practice from a caring base will advance the vital relationship between patient and nurse. Such an emphasis fosters a sense of "feeling cared for" from which safe and quality health outcomes can flourish.

According to Ponte et al. (2007), professionals who acknowledge their unique role, commit to continuous learning, demonstrate professional demeanor, and strive to be inspirational enjoy the benefits of a powerful practice. Taking the risk to renew the commitment to caring and center nursing practice on relationships offers the high road toward an influential practice that will prevail.

SUMMARY

In this chapter, the far-reaching crisis of health care quality has been reviewed. Of particular concern is the slow progress toward its improvement despite the added attention by research and accreditation agencies. Health care quality in the United States has declined in value over the years, and many are in disagreement about its future. Professional nursing, the major health care discipline, is increasingly perceived as less engaged with those they care for; in fact, regularly missed nursing care was described and rationalized in one study, and noncaring nursing behaviors have been detailed since the 1980s. Reporting of nursing-sensitive health care indicators has assisted in generating evidence of nurse quality, and recently, reimbursement systems (Medicare) have added some of them to their incentive procedures. It is only a matter of time until other payors do the same. Professional nursing is in a position to significantly impact the health care system. Through relationship-centered practice, education, and leadership, the amount of time spent in caring interactions can profoundly benefit the quality and safety of American health care.

CALLS TO ACTION

Nursing's future is dependent on a spirit of caring inquiry—practicing from its caring base while simultaneously grounding it in empirical evidence. **Notice** what you are doing and what you are NOT doing.

Reflective Questions/Applications for Students

1. What is your perception of nurse quality?
2. Discuss the state of quality in your health care institution.
3. Are there opportunities for missed nursing care in your institution? What are they? How can these missed opportunities be embraced by the nursing staff?
4. Does professional nursing remain a significant force in today's health care system? How?
5. Describe a noncaring nursing situation you have encountered. What happened? How did you react? What would you do now given the same situation?
6. What nursing-sensitive quality indicators does your organization report? Who is responsible for data collection? Analysis? Report dissemination? Use in practice?
7. Define participatory action research.

Reflective Questions/Applications for Nurse Educators

8. What is values-based learning?
9. What nursing educational research is being conducted at your university?
10. Reflect on the nature of student-faculty relationships at your university. How does it inform your teaching?

11. What learning outcomes are regularly reported by your university? How are they used to refine curricula?

12. How do you assess caring competence in nursing students?

Reflective Questions/Applications for Nurse Leaders

13. How would you rate nursing quality at your institution?

14. What must be implemented at your facility to ensure that RNs spend more time in direct patient care? How would you start? Who would you include?

15. What career development activities/programs are utilized at your institution to recognize and renew nursing's caring core?

REFERENCES

Aiken, L. (2005a). Improving patient safety: The link between nursing and quality of care. *The Robert Wood Johnson Foundation, research in profile.* New Brunswick, NJ: National Program Office.

Aiken, L. H. (2005b). Improving quality through nursing. Improving health and the health care of all Americans. In D. Mechanic, L. Rogut, D. Colby, & J. Knickman (Eds.), *Policy challenges in modern health care.* New Brunswick, NJ: Rutgers University Press.

Aiken, L. H., Clarke, S. P., Cheung, R. B., Sloane, D. M., & Silber, J. H. (2003). Educational levels of hospital nurses and surgical patient mortality. *Journal of the American Medical Association, 290*(12), 1617–1623.

Aiken, L. H., Clarke, S. P., & Sloane, D. M. (2002a). Hospital staffing, organization, and quality of care: Cross national findings. *International Journal of Quality Health Care, 14,* 5–13.

Aiken, L. H., Clarke, S. P., & Sloane, D. M. (2002b). Hospital nurse staffing and patient mortality, nurse burnout, and job dissatisfaction. *Journal of the American Medical Association, 288,* 1987–1993.

Aiken, L. H., Sochalski, J., & Lake, E. T. (1997). Studying outcomes of organizational change in health services. *Medical Care, 35*(11, Suppl.), 6–18.

Amendolair, D. (2008). *Caring behaviors and job satisfaction: Medical surgical nurses, North and South Carolina.* Chapel Hill, NC: 30th Annual International Association for Human Caring.

American Nurses Association (ANA). (1995). *Nursing care report card for acute care.* Washington, DC: Author.

American Nurses Association (ANA). (2000). *NDNQI: Transforming data into quality care.* Retrieved December 5, 2007, from http://www.nursingworld.org/Main MenurCategories/ThePracticeofProfessionalNursing/PatientSafetyQuality/NDNQI/ NDNQI 1NDNQIBrochure.asps

Asch, S. M., Kerr, E. A., Keesey, J., Adams, J. L., Setodji, C. M., Malik, S., et al. (2006). Who is at greatest risk for receiving poor-quality health care? *The New England Journal of Medicine, 354*(11), 1147–1156.

Associated Press. (2007a). *Government outs worst nursing homes.* Retrieved December 4, 2007, from http://www.usatoday.com/news/washington/2007-11-29-nursinghomes_N.htm

Associated Press. (2007b). *R.I. Hospital fined for third instance of doctors operating on wrong side of patient's head.* Retrieved December 4, 2007, from http://www.foxnews.com/story/0,2933,313002,00.html

Attree, M. (2001). Patients' and relatives' experiences and perspectives of 'good' and 'not so good' quality care. *Journal of Advanced Nursing, 33,* 456–466.

Beck, G. (2008). *Hospitals gone bad.* Retrieved January 7, 2008, from http://www.glenbeck.com/content/articles/article/198/3502/

Benner, P., & Wrubel, J (1989). *The primacy of caring: Stress and coping in health and illness.* Menlo Park, CA: Addison-Wesley.

Beurhaus, P., Donelan, K., Ulrich, B., Norman, L., & Dittus, R. (2005). Is the shortage of hospital registered nurses getting better or worse? Findings from two recent national surveys of RNs. *Nursing Economics, 23*(2), 61–71, 96.

Bikker, A. P., & Thompson, A.G.H. (2006). Predicting and comparing patient satisfaction in four different modes of healthcare across a nation. *Social Sciences and Medicine, 63,* 1671–1683.

Boykin, A., & Schoenhofer, S. O. (1993). *Nursing as caring: A model for transforming practice.* New York: National League of Nursing Publications.

Brooten, D., Brooks, L., Madigan, E. A., & Youngblut, J. M. (1998). Home care of high risk pregnant women by advanced practice nurses: Nurse time consumed. *Home Healthcare Nurse, 16,* 823–830.

Brooten, D., Youngblut, J. M., Brown, L., Finkler, S. A., Neff, D. F., & Madigan, E. A. (2001). A randomized trial of nurse specialist home care for women with high-risk pregnancies: Outcomes and costs. *American Journal of Managed Care, 7,* 793–803.

Brooten, D., Youngblut, J. M., Deatrick, J., Naylor, M., & York, R. (2003). APN interventions, time, and contacts using APN transitional care across 5 patient groups. *Journal of Nursing Scholarship, 35,* 73–79.

Brooten, D., Youngblut, J. M., Kutcher, J., & Bobo, C. (2004). Quality and the nursing workforce: APNs, patient outcomes, and health care costs. *Nursing Outlook, 52*(1), 45–52.

Bulman, C., & Schutz, S. (2004). *Reflective practice in nursing.* Boston: Blackwell Publishing.

Burt, K. (2007). *The relationship between nurse caring and selected outcomes of care in hospitalized older adults.* Unpublished doctoral dissertation, The Catholic University of America.

Chang, B. L., Lee, J. L., Peason, M. L., Kahn, K. L., Elliott, M. N., & Rubenstein, L. L. (2002). Evaluating quality of nursing care: The gap between theory and practice. *Journal of Nursing Administration, 32*(7/8), 405–418.

Clancy, C. M., Farquhar, B., & Sharp, B.A.C. (2005). Patient safety in nursing practice. *Journal of Nursing Care Quality, 20*(3), 193–197.

Consumer Reports. (2003). *How safe is your hospital?* Retrieved December 4, 2007, from http://www.consumerreports.org/cro/health-fitness/health-care/hospitals-how safe-103/overview/

Corchado, A., & Iliff, L. (2007, July 30). U.S. patients choosing Mexican hospitals for price, quality. *The Dallas Morning News,* p. 3.

Davis, K., Schoen, C., Schoenbaum, S., Doty, M. M., Holgren, A. S., Kriss, J. L., et al. (2004). *Mirror, mirror on the wall: An international update on the comparative performance of American health care.* New York: The Commonwealth Fund.

Dingman, S., Williams, M., Fosbinder, D., & Warnnick, M. (1999). Implementing a caring model to improve patient satisfaction. *Journal of Nursing Administration, 29*(12), 630–638.

Donabedian, A. (1966). Evaluating the quality of medical care. *Milbank Memorial Fund Quarterly: Health and Society, 44*(3, Pt. 2), 166–203.

Dunton, N., Grajewski, B., Taunton, R. L., & Moore, J. (2004). Nurse staffing and patient falls on acute care hospital units. *Nursing Outlook, 52*(1), 53–59.

Duffy, J. (1992). The impact of nurse caring on patient outcomes. In D. Gaut (Ed.), *The presence of caring in nursing.* New York: National League for Nursing Press.

Duffy, J. (2005). Want to graduate nurses who care? Assessing nursing students' caring competencies. *Annual Review of Nursing Education, 3,* 73–97.

Duffy, J., Baldwin, J., & Mastorovich, M. J. (2007).Using the Quality-Caring Model© to organize patient care. *Journal of Nursing Administration, 37*(12), 546–551.

Duffy, J., & Hoskins, L. (2003). The Quality-Caring Model©: Blending dual paradigms. *Advances in Nursing Science, 26*(1), 77–88.

Fagin, C. (2001). *When care becomes a burden: Diminishing access to adequate nursing.* The Milbank Memorial Fund. Retrieved October 5, 2007, from http://www.milbank.org/reports/01026fagin.html

Florin, J., Ehrenberg, A., & Ehnfors, M. (2005). Patients' and nurses' perceptions of nursing problems in an acute care setting. *Journal of Advanced Nursing, 51*(2), 140–149.

Gallagher, R. M. (2005). National quality efforts: What continuing and staff development educators need to know. *The Journal of Continuing Education in Nursing, 36*(1), 40–45.

Gallagher, R. M., & Rowell, P. A. (2003). Claiming the future of nursing through nursing-sensitive quality indicators. *Nursing Administration Quarterly, 27*(4), 273–284.

General Accounting Office. (2003, July). *Nursing home quality,* GAO-03-561. Washington, DC: Author.

Health Grades, Inc. (2007). *The Tenth Annual Health Grades Hospital Quality in America Study.* Retrieved October 29, 2007, from http://www.healthgrades.com

Hendrickson, G., Doddato, T. M., & Kovner, C. T. (1990). How do nurses use their time? *Journal of Nursing Administration, 20*(3), 31–38.

Hughes, R., & Clancy, C. (2007). Improving the complex nature of care transitions. *Journal of Nursing Care Quality, 22*(4), 289–292.

Institute for Healthcare Improvement. (2007). *Transforming care at the bedside. Joint Commission on Accreditation of Health Care Organizations. Improving America's Hospitals: The Joint Commission's annual report on quality and safety 2007.* Retrieved December 4, 2007, from http://www.jointcommissionreport.org/executive/executivesummary.aspx

Institute of Medicine (IOM). (1999). *To err is human: Building a safer health system.* Washington, DC: National Academy Press.

Institute of Medicine (IOM). (2001). *Crossing the quality chasm: A new health system for the 21st century.* Committee on Quality of Health Care in America. Washington, DC: National Academy Press.

Joint Commission for Accreditation of Healthcare Organizations. (2007). *Improving America's hospitals. The Joint Commission's annual report on quality and safety.* Retrieved January 6, 2008, from http://www.jointcommissionreport.org/

Kalisch, B. J. (2006). Missed nursing care: A qualitative study. *Journal of Nursing Care Quality, 21*(4), 306–313.

Kelly, L. (1988). The ethic of caring: Has it been discarded? *Nursing Outlook, 36*(1), 48.

Klevens, M. R., Edwards, J. R., Richards, C. L., Horan, T. C., Gaynes, R. P., Pollock, D. A., et al. (2007). Estimating health care-associated infections and deaths in US hospitals, 2002. *Public Health Reports, 122,* 160–166.

Kowalczyk, L. (2007, March 17). Surprise check faults MGH quality of care. *The Boston Globe.*

Kurtzman, E. T., & Corrigan, J. M. (2007). Measuring the contribution of nursing to quality, patient safety, and health care outcomes. *Policy, Politics, & Nursing Practice, 8*(1), 20–25.

Lang, N. (2003). Reflections on quality health care. *Nursing Administration Quarterly, 27*(4), 266–272.

Latham, C. P. (1996). Predictors of patient outcomes following interactions with nurses. *Western Journal of Nursing Research, 18*(5), 548–564.

Leininger, M. (1998). Culture care: Diversity and universality theory. In A. M. Tomey & M. R. Alligood (Eds.), *Nursing theorists and their work* (4th ed., pp. 439–462). St. Louis, MO: Mosby.

Linden, L., & English, K. (1994). Adjusting the cost-quality equation: Utilizing work sampling and time study data to redesign clinical practice. *Journal of Nursing Care Quality, 8*(3), 34–42.

Lynn, M. R., McMillen, B. J. & Sidana, S. (2007). Understanding and measuring patients' assessment of the quality of nursing care. *Nursing Research, 56*(3), 159–166.

Muntlin, A., Gunningberg, L., & Carlsson, M. (2006). Patients' perceptions of quality of care at an emergency department and identification of areas for quality improvement. *Journal of Clinical Nursing, 15,* 1045–1056.

National League for Nursing. (2007). *Task group on funding for nursing education research final report.* New York: Author.

National Quality Forum. (2004). *National voluntary consensus standards for nursing-sensitive care: An initial performance measure set.* Washington, DC: Author.

Naylor, M. (2003). Nursing intervention research and quality of care: Influencing the future of healthcare. *Nursing Research, 52*(6), 380–385.

Naylor, M., Brooten, D., Campbell, R., Jacobsen, B., Mezey, M., Pauley, M., et al. (1999). Comprehensive discharge planning and home follow-up of hospitalized elders: A randomized controlled trial. *Journal of the American Medical Association, 281,* 613–620.

Needleman, J., & Buerhaus, P. I. (2003). Nurse staffing and patient safety: Current knowledge and implications for actions. *International Journal of Quality Health Care, 15,* 275–277.

Needleman, J., Buerhaus, P. I., Mattke, S., Stewart, M., & Zelevinsky, K. (2002). Nurse staffing levels and quality of care in hospitals. *New England Journal of Medicine, 346,* 1415–1422.

Ponte, P. R., Glazer, G., Dann, E., McCollum, K., Gross, A., Tyrrell, R., et al. (2007). The power of professional nursing practice. *Online Journal of Issues in Nursing,*

12(1). Retrieved October 2, 2007, from http://www.nursingworld.org/MainMenu Categories/ANAMarketplace/ANAPeriodicals/OJIN/TableofContents/Volume 122007/No1Jan07/tpc32_316092.aspx

Proudfoot, M. (1983). Contagious calmness: A sense of calmness in acute care settings. *Topics in Clinical Nursing, 5,* 18–29.

Pullen, R. L., Murray, P. H., & McGee, K. S. (2001). Care groups: A model to mentor novice nursing students. *Nurse Educator, 26*(6), 283–288.

Reiman, D. J. (1986). Non-caring and caring in the clinical setting. *Topics in Clinical Nursing, 8,* 30–36.

Roach, M. S. (1984). *Caring the human mode of being, implications for nursing.* Toronto: University of Toronto.

Robert Wood Johnson Foundation. (2006, March). All Americans at risk of receiving poor quality health care. *RWJF Research Highlight, 1.*

Robert Wood Johnson Foundation (RWJF). (2007). *CMS rule limiting payment for avoidable complications has big implications for nurses.* Retrieved December 4, 2007, from http://www.rwjf.org/programareas/resources/product.jsp?id=23434&pid=1142&gsa=1

Rogers, A. E., Hwang, W. T., Scott, L. D., Aiken, L. H., & Dinges, D. F. (2004). The working hours of hospital staff nurses and patient safety. *Health Affairs, 23*(4), 202–212.

Rutherford, P., Lee, B., & Greiner, A. (2004). *Transforming care at the bedside.* IHI Innovation Series white paper. Boston: Institute for Healthcare Improvement (Available on http://www.IHI.org).

Schaffer, M. A., & Juarez, M. (1996). A strategy to enhance caring and community in the learning environment. *Nurse Educator, 21*(5), 43–47.

Simpson, R. (2008). Caring communications: How technology enhances interpersonal relations, part 1. *Nursing Administration Quarterly, 32*(1), 70–73.

Sochalski, J. (2004). Is more better? The relationship between nurse staffing and the quality of nursing care in hospitals. *Medical Care, 42*(2, Suppl.), II-67–II-73.

Swan, B. (1998). Postoperative nursing care contributions to symptom distress and functional status after ambulatory surgery. *MEDSURG Nursing, 7*(3), 148–158.

Swanson, K. M. (1991). Empirical development of a middle range theory of caring. *Nursing Research, 40*(3), 161–166.

Thorsteinsson, L. (2002). The quality of nursing care as perceived by individuals with chronic illnesses: The magical touch of nursing. *Journal of Clinical Nursing, 11*(1), 32–40.

Todaro-Franceschi, V. (2007). Imagining nursing practice in the year 2050: Looking through a Rogerian looking glass. *Nursing Science Quarterly, 20*(3), 229–231.

Trafford, A. (2001, January 7). When the hospital staff isn't enough. *Washington Post,* A01.

Trzeciak, S., & Rivers, E. P. (2003). Emergency department overcrowding in the United States: An emerging threat to patient safety and public health. *Journal of Emergency Medicine, 20,* 402–405.

Urden, L. D., & Roode, J. L. (1997). Work sampling: A decision-making tool for determining resources and work redesign. *Journal of Nursing Administration, 27*(9), 34–41.

Vahey, D. C., Aiken, L. H., Sloane, D. M., Clarke, S. P., & Vargas, D. (2004). Nurse burnout and patient satisfaction. *Medical Care, 42*(2, Suppl.), II-57–II-66.

Watson, J. (1979). *Nursing: The philosophy and science of caring.* Boston: Little, Brown and Company.

Watson, J. (1985). *Nursing: Human science and human care.* Norwalk, CT: Appleton-Century-Crofts.

Watson, J. (2006). Caring theory as ethical guide to administrative and clinical practices. *Journal of Nursing Administration, 8*(1), 87–93.

Wolf, Z. R., Colahan, M., & Costello, A. (1998). Relationship between nurse caring and patient satisfaction. *MEDSURG Nursing, 7*(2), 99–105.

Yeakel, S., Maljanian, R., Bohannon, R. W., & Coulombe, K. (2003). Nurse caring behaviors and patient satisfaction: Improvement after a multifaceted staff intervention. *Journal of Nursing Administration, 33*(9), 434–436.

A Framework for Quality Nursing Practice

Relationships are where it all comes together . . . or comes apart.
—Philip Crosby

Keywords: nursing theory, caring, relationships

PHILOSOPHICAL AND THEORETICAL UNDERPINNINGS

In general, the word *quality* has connotations of superiority and excellence. It represents a characteristic or attribute of a service or product that demonstrates its worth. Quality of products and services has a long history dating back to the middle ages where groups of skilled craftsmen organized in guilds to ensure standards were met (History Learning Site, 2008). During World War II, the quality of products manufactured in the United States, particularly related to ammunition, became an important priority. Emphasis on quality continued as the Japanese used the input of W. Edwards Deming (1966, 1986, 2000) and Joseph M. Juran (2003; Juran & Godfrey, 1999) to incite a quality revolution that eventually became noticed by the U.S. industrial sector. Utilizing statistical techniques, strong leadership, and process improvement, American companies gradually embraced the concept of total quality management (TQM; Williams, 1994). The term *total quality management* has evolved to *performance improvement* (PI) and is now a routine component of all industries including nonprofits such as governments, education, and health care.

In health care, quality has been defined as "the degree to which health services . . . increase the likelihood of desired health outcomes and are consistent with current professional knowledge" (Lohr, et al., 1990). Furthermore, health care is considered to be of a high quality "when it is safe, effective, patient-centered, timely, efficient, and equitable" (Naylor, 2003, p. 381). Dr. Avedis Donabedian, considered the father of health care quality, provided the health care community with a definition and theoretical framework for quality that continues to provide the foundation for performance improvement activities today (Donabedian, 1966, 1980, 1986, 1992). In his notion of expert health care, quality included scientific or technical aspects as well as interpersonal aspects. The three major components of his framework include: structure, process, and outcomes. *Structure* refers to the context or conditions under which care is provided. Factors such as institutional resources, organizational culture, provider credentials, and patient characteristics comprise this component. *Process* refers to activities done for the patient, including both the technical and interpersonal aspects of care (Donabedian, 1980). Specific interventions and activities based on appropriate standards and evidence-based guidelines, as well as interpersonal aspects of care, are included in the process of care component. *Outcomes* refer to the consequences of the health care process including clinical parameters and patient perceptions of the experience, such as patient satisfaction. This framework has been and continues to be the basis for the Joint Commission on Accreditation of Healthcare Organizations' (JCAHO) review process.

Dr. Norma Lang (1976) introduced a nursing approach to measuring quality that included the formation of values informed by society, professional beliefs, and scientific knowledge. Next, criteria for nursing care standards were established. Measuring the degree of discrepancy between the standards and criteria and the current level of nursing practice was then evaluated. Revising or improving nursing care based on the data completed the process. Dr. Lang also advocated for a standardized language for nursing so measuring and improving care could be compared across settings in an efficient manner.

In 1998, Mitchell, Ferketich, and Jennings, members of the American Academy of Nursing's (AAN) Expert Panel on Quality Health Care, criticized Donabedian's (1966) structure, process, and outcomes framework as too linear and offered a more vibrant approach toward understanding quality health care. In their model, recognition of the dynamic reciprocal relationships between the system, intervention, client, and outcome components is explicated. Thus, interventions are mediated by client and system characteristics and outcomes are influenced by and interact with all the variables.

With a more nursing-oriented slant, Irvine, Sidani, and McGillis Hall (1998) developed the Nursing Role Effectiveness Model based on Donabedian's earlier work, with the addition of nursing-specific roles. In this model, the independent, dependent, and interdependent roles of nurses are clarified highlighting the contribution of nursing to health care outcomes.

Nursing's theoretical/philosophical pioneers also provide some foundational context for quality. Many spoke to nursing quality in terms of improving patients' health. In particular, Nightingale (1859) viewed nursing as crucial to the health and safety of its recipients. Nightingale was committed to her patients' needs and relentless in her approach to quality health care. She searched for "root causes" and led improvements in efficiency. Although not known as such at the time, Nightingale role-modeled evidence-based practice, by collecting data and compiling statistics for use in improving the health care of her patients (Meyer & Bishop, 2007). Then, using her findings, she presented mortality data to her superiors as the basis for revisions in services.

Most nursing theorists speak to quality as an important aspect of nursing. Although not included as a metaparadigm concept per se, quality is an implicit concept common to many nursing theories. It is most often related to the concept of *health,* one of the metaparadigm concepts. *Health* is patient-defined and connotes well-being, comfort, holism, and optimal functioning. Based on the theorist, there is often an intermediate objective that contributes to health, such as coping, adaptation, self-care, transactions, or feeling cared for. Furthermore, the role of the nurse as stated in various nursing theories speaks to "assisting, interacting, intervening, advocating, and educating" all in an effort to promote health (King, 1981; Orem, 2001; Peplau, 1988; Roy, 1980; Travelbee, 1966). Interestingly, a common theme among many nursing theorists is the therapeutic characteristics of nursing, particularly the nurse–patient relationship. In fact, Chinn and Kramer (2004) describe human interaction as the primary focus of nursing that distinguishes it from other health care disciplines.

RELATIONSHIPS AND HEALTH CARE

It is through relationships that individuals live, learn, work, change, and grow beginning in the earliest stages of life. Such relationships exist in one dimension with other humans, such as family members and friends, as well as with nonhumans, such as pets or the environment. Some might say another form of relationship exists in a higher dimension that is spiritual or universal. Relationships are complex, nonlinear experiences that mature over time. Relationships are unique to persons and throughout life function as points of reference; thus, relationships become supportive to persons so much so that often they go unnoticed. During the health/illness continuum, relationships continue to be required to meet the human challenges of uncertainty, finding meaning, financial and social welfare, dependency, lifestyle changes, and modification of social roles. But as all too many people who are hospitalized know, loved ones are often precluded from visiting and participating in care decisions, leaving them to bear their difficulties in lonely isolation. As early as 1994, researchers studying the effects of personal connections on health called attention to the healing effects of family and friends' visitation on hospitalized patients (Cohen, Kaplan, & Manuck, 1994).

Research is beginning to demonstrate that relational variables are important in improving health care outcomes. Evidence concerning the link between relationships and physical health has established that people with deep personal connections—that is, who are married, have close family and friends, are active in social and religious groups—recover more quickly from disease and live longer. A case in point is the study on relationship stress and the healing ability of the human body (Kiecolt-Glaser, et al., 2005).

In this study of 42 married couples, the researchers focused on those who had been together an average of at least 12 years. Each couple was admitted into the university's clinical research center for two, 24-hour visits. The visits were separated by a two-month interval. At the beginning of the study, the subjects completed questionnaires to assess their stress levels. During each visit, both the husband and wife were fitted with suction devices that created eight identical blisters on their arms. The skin was removed from each blister and another device placed directly over each small wound, forming a protective bubble, from which researchers could extract the fluids that normally fill such blisters. And finally, each subject had a catheter inserted through which blood could be drawn for analysis.

During the first visit, each spouse was asked to talk for several minutes about some characteristic or behavior that he or she would like to change. This was a supportive, positive discussion. At the second visit, however, the subjects were asked to talk about an area of disagreement. This typically was a topic that was emotionally charged. Both discussions were videotaped, and those tapes were used to gauge the level of hostility present between the couples. Fluid accumulating at the individual wound sites and peripheral blood samples were also taken from each participant. The study results showed that wounds took a day longer to heal after the arguments than they did after the initial supportive discussion; and couples who showed high levels of hostility needed two days longer for wound-healing compared to couples whose hostility appeared low. Blood samples from those highly hostile couples showed differences as well. The levels of one cytokine—interleukin-6 (IL-6)—increased one-and-a-half times over those in couples considered less hostile. The fact that a simple marital disagreement could delay healing for a day was a profound finding in this study.

In another study, marital quality and survival from heart failure were investigated. Patients who had more negative relationships with their spouses were 1.8 times as likely to die within 4 years compared to those who had less negative ratings (Coyne, Rohrbaugh, Shoham, & Sonnega, 2001). In addition to marital relationships, individuals who had ongoing religious/spirituality practices were found to have better health outcomes, including less pain (Rippentrop, Altmaier, Chen, Found, & Keffala, 2005). At the National Center for Complementary and Alternative Medicine (NCCAM), a part of the National Institutes of Health, funded projects on body–mind connections have "focused on the interactions among the brain, mind, body, and behavior, and on the powerful ways in which emotional, mental, social, spiritual, and behavioral factors can directly affect health. It regards as fundamental an approach that respects and enhances each person's capacity for self-knowledge and self-care, and it emphasizes techniques that are grounded in this approach" (NCCAM, 2007).

In 1994, the Fetzer Institution, a private foundation, in partnership with the Pew Charitable Trust, published a document titled *Relationship-Centered Care* (Tresolini, 1994) in which an integrated approach to health professional curricula was examined. In this monograph, relationships as the central component of health care were acknowledged. Interestingly, it was noted that "despite nursing's long history emphasizing caring relationships in its practice and ethos, this focus has not become a defining force in health care" (p. 11). So, to forge a reformed health care future, the task force developed a health care curriculum that was founded on several important relationships: (1) patient–practitioner relationships, (2) community–practitioner relationships, and (3) practitioner–practitioner relationships. Knowledge and skills in self-awareness and continuing self-growth, the patient's experience of health and illness, developing and maintaining relationships with patients, and communicating clearly and effectively were considered crucial. As a result of this work, the Indiana University School of Medicine (2005) began a three-year process in January 2003 of self-study and organizational development known as the Relationship-Centered Care Initiative (RCCI). They restructured the medical curriculum around relationships and have gone on to provide workshops for others interested in educating physicians this way (Indiana University School of Medicine, 2005). Finally, in the Institute of Medicine (IOM) report, *Crossing the Quality Chasm* (2001), "care based on continuous, healing relationships" was listed as the first rule of redesign for the fractured health care system of today (p. 61).

The foundation for care provided by health professionals is the personal relationship between the clinician and the patient. It is through this relationship that information is exchanged, feelings and concerns are shared, interventions are provided, and outcomes are attained. For nursing, it has been cited as a moral imperative (Hartman, 1998). Recently, Suchman (2006) offered theoretical support for shared relationships in health care by discussing the *complex responsive processes of relating* (CRPR), a new theoretical perspective on human interaction. Drawing on complexity theory (Stacey, 2001), patterns of meaning and relating are continuously formed through ongoing reciprocal interactions; these multifaceted, nonlinear patterns are self-organizing and over time result in emerging new patterns.

In this light, a health care organization is a complex system composed of several smaller complex systems, such as individual units or departments and the people, structures, and processes who compose them. There is no outside control in a complex system (hence no need for hierarchy) because the multiple interdependent interactions "teach" the system how to adapt to changing conditions. This repetitive sequence of taking in and then doing enables the system to self-advance. The attention to and quality of relationships in complex systems are keys to progression.

Relationships among health care professionals caring for specific patients have also been demonstrated to be associated with improved health outcomes (Brewer, 2006). Safran, Miller, and Beckman (2006) described seven qualities essential for "interdependent and mutually reinforcing" (p. S11) collaborative relationships. They are: mindfulness, diversity of mental models, heedful interrelating, a mix of rich and lean communication, a mix of social and task-related interactions, mutual respect, and trust. In this paper, Safran et al. (2006) present empirical evidence for such relationships as essential to specific patient (reduced mortality, improved functional health), system (decreased lengths of stay), and provider (workforce moral and turnover) outcomes.

As the mounting evidence is suggesting the importance of relationships to quality of care, the health care system is beginning to notice, and nursing, in particular, has renewed its interest in *caring relationships* as the essence of its profession. The Quality-Caring Model© places relationships at the heart of the health care process, particularly the caring relationships that are integral to nursing practice (Duffy & Hoskins, 2003). It speculates that caring relationships not only improve patient care but also advance nurses' individual and collective professional growth.

DEFINITIONS, CONCEPTS, AND ASSUMPTIONS OF THE QUALITY-CARING MODEL

Assumptions are beliefs we hold to be true based on any number of cultural, biological, intellectual, and experiential influences. That being said, the assumptions related to the Quality-Caring Model center around the critical components of *participants, caring relationships, feeling "cared for," and health.* The participants in this model are the individuals included in the health care experience and can be identified as patients, providers, or the system (the organization) itself. Individuals are inherently worthy and function "in relationship" to others. They are biopsychossocioculturalspiritual beings who have characteristics (certain descriptive features), attitudes and behaviors, and life experiences that are unique. The whole of an individual's characteristics, attitudes and behaviors, and

Stoxen Library Dickinson State Univ

life experiences provide the basis for a phenomenal field that releases energy and is continually interacting and changing with the environment (Rogers, 1961). Individuals' subjective reality or phenomenal field influences the meaning of their experiences, including health and illness.

Caring relationships are human interactions grounded in caring factors. They are nonlinear and characterized by mutuality among the participants. Caring relationships comprise specific activities (doing) as well as specific attitudes (being with).

Assumptions about caring relationships include:

- Caring relationships are essential for well-being and growth
- Interaction is necessary for caring relationships
- Caring relationships are grounded in beliefs about individuals
- Caring relationships consist of factors or processes
- Caring relationships are tangible and can be measured
- Caring relationships are essential to the practice of nursing
- Caring relationships require knowledge, self-awareness, and skill

A consequence of caring relationships as espoused in the Quality-Caring Model is feeling "cared for." This emotion is important because it is associated with contentment, met needs, acceptance, and validation (Mashek & Aron, 2004). As individuals perceive being "cared for" by their health care providers, they experience ease, protection from harm, and maintenance of their human dignity. In this state, "a sense of security develops that makes it easier to learn new things, change behaviors, take risks, and follow guidelines" (Duffy & Hoskins, 2003, p. 83). Assumptions about feeling "cared for" are:

- Feeling "cared for" is a positive concept
- Feeling "cared for" occurs as a result of caring interaction/s
- Feeling "cared for" is desired by recipients of the health care process

Assumptions concerning health in the Quality-Caring Model focus on its multidimensional nature, which, when attained, connotes quality. Health is generally considered a positive concept that is regarded as valuable by society. While society deems health to be valuable, it is defined at the individual level as a more subjective and holistic perception that influences how an individual interacts

(continued)

with his/her environment and uncovers meaning in his/her life. In this model, health refers to all participants including patients, providers, and systems.

Some assumptions about health include:

- Health is dynamic
- Health is a state of physical, emotional, and spiritual integration
- Health is contextual

THE QUALITY-CARING MODEL

The Quality-Caring Model (see Figure 2.1) was developed in 2003 to "preserve the essence of nursing within the realities of modern healthcare" (Duffy & Hoskins, 2003). It was designed as a middle-range theory to support the understanding of the connections between quality health care and caring. As a middle-range theory, it seeks to describe and explain concepts important to quality health care as well as to guide research. Most importantly, however, it was intended to support nursing by focusing on the important caring relationships that undergird its practice.

The Quality-Caring Model evolved over time and was built on the work of others. Through deductive processes, research, and borrowing from the disciplines of medicine, sociology, and psychology the model explains how nursing links to quality. It is grounded in the works of Donabedian (1966) and Watson (1979, 1985) and influenced by contributions from King (1981), Mitchell et al. (1998), and Irvine et al. (1998).

The Quality-Caring Model integrates biomedical and psychosociocultural spiritual factors associated with quality health care. It specifies the types and attributes of relationships that contribute to quality health care. Thus, the major concepts are measurable and can be empirically validated. The major proposition of the model is that caring relationships influence attainment of positive health outcomes for patients/families, health care providers, and health care systems (Duffy & Hoskins, 2003). Inherent in the model is the continuous search for evidence of quality.

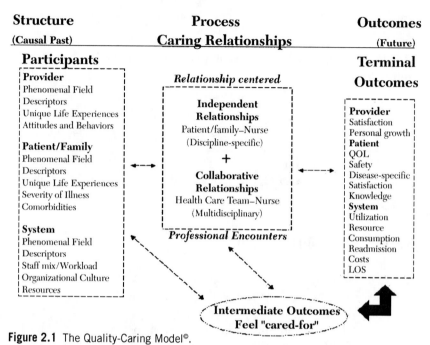

Figure 2.1 The Quality-Caring Model©.

From "The Quality-Caring Model©: Blending Dual Paradigms," by J. Duffy and L. M. Hoskins, 2003, *Advances in Nursing Science, 26*(1), 77–88.

The first main construct, *structure,* refers to the composition of individuals or systems (participants) involved in delivering quality health care. For this purpose, patients, providers, and the system itself are highlighted. Each are inherently worthy and have unique characteristics and life experiences that together comprise their "phenomenal field" or subjective reality. Patients are those individuals who have health care needs and have attributes such as specific demographics, severity of illness, and comorbidities that can influence both the processes and outcomes of health care. Providers have unique characteristics such as credentials, attitudes, and behaviors that can affect the processes of care and, indirectly, health care outcomes. Regarding the health care system, characteristics such as resources, organizational culture, and others unique to the setting are subconcepts.

Process of care, the second major construct, is the main focus of this model. The process of care is relationship-centered and grounded in caring factors. Although these factors were initially theorized to be grounded in Watson's 10 Carative Factors (1979, 1985), recent evidence suggests that 8 caring factors comprise caring relationships (Duffy, Hoskins, & Seifert, 2007). Examples of these factors include mutual problem solving, such as negotiating the living arrangements of an elderly relative or attending to human needs by gently providing mouth care to a ventilator-dependent patient. (See Table 2.1 for a complete list of caring factors.)

Using the caring factors as the foundation for nursing practice ensures that professional encounters are of a caring nature.

Caring relationships emphasize reverence for persons and the meanings associated with health and illness. The ability of professional nurses to put themselves in another's context, to perceive their way of being in the world is the fundamental nature of caring relationships.

King (1981) called this phenomenon *perceptual accuracy,* which is a process that requires knowledge that may not come naturally. Through human interaction, nurses choose to recognize persons in need of health care, view them as unique individuals with preferences who can make

Table 2.1

EIGHT CARING FACTORS

Mutual problem solving

Attentive reassurance

Human respect

Encouraging manner

Appreciation of unique meanings

Healing environment

Affiliation needs

Basic human needs

From "Dimension of Caring: Psychometric Evaluation of the Caring Assessment Tool," by J. Duffy, L. M. Hoskins, and R. F. Seifert, 2007, *Advances in Nursing Science, 30*(3), 235–245.

appropriate decisions, and use interventions in a caring manner that are known to be beneficial.

In the Quality-Caring Model, the caring relationships that are established with patients and families are independent functions of nurses. Included are those attitudes and behaviors that nurses implement autonomously and are solely held accountable for. Independent relationships facilitate discipline-specific interventions, such as managing pain, and lead to nursing-sensitive patient outcomes. They may affect other outcomes of care as well. Specific caring factors should be used to guide the nurse as he/she assists the patient and family. It is through such relationships that outcomes such as increased knowledge, safety, comfort, adherence, and anxiety may be affected. Within the independent patient/family–nurse relationship, the focus is on the needs of patients and their families. Yet, feelings of being "cared for" can also occur and affect the nurse.

Both independent (discipline-specific) relationships as well as collaborative (interprofessional) relationships comprise the concept, relationship-centered professional encounters. Collaborative relationships include those activities and responsibilities that nurses share with other members of the health care team. Such relationships are shared, and all the professionals working together in unity form a new relationship that is collectively more than the sum of the individuals. This new relationship would be characterized by Watson (1979, 1985) as transpersonal, that is, a shared experience that creates its own phenomenal field. Research in the aviation industry has consistently demonstrated that the way professionals work together for a common purpose has a profound impact on outcomes (Thomas, Sherwood, and Helmreich, 2003). In fact, airline safety measured as accident rates has remained relatively constant over the last two decades despite increased traffic and worldwide travel. In the health care industry, the national Acute Physiology and Chronic Health Evaluation (APACHE) study found that the distinguishing feature between hospitals with exceptional outcomes from intensive care and those with poor outcomes was the collaborative working relationship between the nurses and physicians (Knaus, Draper, Wagner, & Zimmerman, 1986).

Interprofessional collaborative relationships are enhanced when mutual partnerships exist among the various professionals focused on the best interests of patients and their families. Nurses' use of caring factors facilitates cooperation and coordination among the varied members of the health care team. Examples of this include viewing all team members as partners with valuable input to share, actively participating during team rounds, facilitating team problem solving, teaching new members, and coordinating care conferences. When teams function cohesively, continuity is maintained and patients and families as well as team members feel "cared for."

To maximize independent and collaborative relationships, nurses must be experts in initiating, cultivating, and sustaining caring relationships. Human caring requires nurses to value and commit to relationship-building. It also requires the capability to conceptualize the whole rather than fragmented parts. Becoming more knowledgeable about clinical caring and demonstrating it in relationships demand the courage to proudly affirm that caring is the dominant focus of nursing. Caring relationships are uniting; they provide the context through which specific interventions are implemented or teams make decisions. While independent relationships with patients and families are primary, collaborative relationships are essential to quality care. Balancing the two relationships in the best interests of the patient and family is outcome-enhancing for the patient, the provider, and the health care system. "The role of the nurse is to be the link between the patient/family, the healthcare team and . . . outcomes" (Duffy & Hoskins, 2003, p. 83). In fact, Duffy and Hoskins (2003) consider it nursing's primary work.

> This blended approach to enhancing health care quality emphasizes the centrality of caring relationships and provides a practical way to generate evidence of its value. The core of this patient-driven model is human beings in relationships; practicing this core may lead to improved health outcomes for patients and families and energized health care professionals who, along with the systems they are working in, are remembering daily why they chose to care.

SUMMARY

This chapter reviewed the concept of *quality*, including its definition and theoretical understanding. The human interactions pertinent to health care are considered influencing factors in quality. Evidence linking relational variables to health care outcomes was described as was the quality of relationships between health care professionals. The Quality-Caring

Model was introduced as a blended framework for improving patient outcomes and advancing professional nursing. Its definitions, concepts, and assumptions were presented, and its description as a middle-range (practical) theory was illustrated. Independent and collaborative relationships inherent in the model were defined and their consequences analyzed. Finally, the role of the professional nurse as the link between patients and families and health care outcomes was emphasized.

CALLS TO ACTION

Noticing the others' perspective or worldview along with appreciating the impact of health and illness on his/her holistic nature is an underlying premise of caring relationships. **Observe** how illness is affecting the physical, emotional, social, cultural, and spiritual dimensions of your next patient.

Building caring relationships starts by valuing the phenomenon of human creation, acquiring knowledge in clinical caring, and then courageously expressing caring through ongoing human connection/s. **Reflect** on the beauty of the human person as he/she lives in relation to the universe.

Reflective Questions/Applications for Students

1. Describe Donabedian's (1966) Quality Medical Care Model; include each of the major concepts.
2. Discuss how nursing's many theorists contributed to the notion of quality health care.
3. Provide at least three sources of evidence for the influence of relationships on health.
4. What are the assumptions and major proposition/s of the Quality-Caring Model?
5. What comprises caring relationships?
6. Describe the independent function of nursing as stated in the Quality-Caring Model.
7. Develop a paper on the "Quality Gurus." Analyze their thoughts and processes of quality and synthesize how their work contributed to the American business world. Then, extrapolate from

their work specific recommendations for health care that can be realistically applied.

8. On the Internet, examine the Fetzer Foundation and University of Indiana School of Medicine's Relationship Centered Caring Initiative (RCCI) Web sites. What activities are identified on these sites that enhance health professionals' knowledge and skills in relationship-building?

Reflective Questions/Applications for Educators

9. How is quality defined in education?
10. What teaching strategies would you use to effectively help students learn about human relationships?
11. Consider the assumption, "Caring relationships are tangible and can be measured." Do you agree or disagree?

Reflective Questions/Applications for Nurse Leaders

12. Reflect on the many interdependent relationships that exist in your complex systems. How do they shape the system?
13. Describe a situation in which you cultivated a caring interprofessional relationship. What happened? What was your role? What did you learn from this experience?

REFERENCES

Brewer, B. (2006). Relationships among teams, culture, safety, and cost outcomes. *Western Journal of Nursing Research, 28*(6), 641–653.

Chinn, P. L., & Kramer, M. K. (2004). *Integrated knowledge development* (6th ed.). St. Louis, MO: CV Mosby.

Cohen, S., Kaplan, J. R., & Manuck, S. B. (1994). Social support and coronary heart disease: Underlying psychologic and biologic mechanisms. In S. A. Shumaker & S. M. Czajkowski (Eds.), *Social support and cardiovascular disease.* New York: Plenum.

Coyne, J. C., Rohrbaugh, M. J., Shoham, J. S., & Sonnega, J. M. (2001). Prognostic importance of marital quality for survival of congestive heart failure. *American Journal of Cardiology, 88,* 526–529.

Deming, W. E. (1966). *Some theory of sampling.* New York: Dover Publications.

Deming, W. E. (1986). *Out of the crisis.* Boston, MA: MIT Press.

Deming, W. E. (2000). *The new economics for industry, government, education* (2nd ed.). Boston, MA: MIT Press.

Donabedian, A. (1966). Evaluating the quality of medical care. *The Milbank Memorial Fund Quarterly, 44*(Pt. 2), 166–203.

Donabedian, A. (1980). Methods for deriving criteria for assessing the quality of care. *Medical Care Review, 37,* 653–698.

Donabedian, A. (1986). Criteria and standards for quality assurance and monitoring. *Quarterly Review Bulletin, 12*, 99–108.

Donabedian, A. (1992). The role of outcomes in quality assessment and assurance. *Quality Review Bulletin, 18*, 356–360.

Duffy, J., & Hoskins, L. (2003). The Quality-Caring Model©: Blending dual paradigms. *Advances in Nursing Science, 26*(1), 77–88.

Duffy, J., Hoskins, L. M., & Seifert, R. F. (2007). Dimensions of caring: Psychometric properties of the Caring Assessment Tool. *Advances in Nursing Science, 30*(3), 235–245.

Hartman, R. L. (1998). Revisiting the call to care: An ethical perspective. *Advanced Practice Nursing Quarterly, 4*(2), 14–18.

History Learning Site. (2008). *Medieval guilds.* Retrieved February 2, 2008, from http://www.historylearningsite.co.uk/medievalguilds.htm

Indiana University School of Medicine. (2005). *The RCCI Newsletter, 2*(1, Winter). Retrieved December 5, 2007, from http://meca.iusm.iu.edu/Resources/RCCI%20Winter%202005%20Newsletter.pdf

Institute of Medicine. (2001). *Crossing the quality chasm: A new health system for the 21st century.* Committee on Quality of Health Care in America. Washington, DC: National Academy Press.

Irvine, D. M., Sidani, S., & McGillis Hall, L. (1998). Linking outcomes to nurses' roles in health care. *Nursing Economics, 16*(2), 58–64.

Juran, J. M. (2003). *Architect of quality.* New York: McGraw-Hill.

Juran, J. M., & Godfrey, A. B. (1999). *Juran's quality handbook.* New York: McGraw-Hill.

Kiecolt-Glaser, J. K., Loving, T. J., Stowell, J. R., Malarkey, W. B., Lemeshow, S., Dickinson, S. L., et al. (2005). Hostile marital interactions, proinflammatory cytokine production, and wound healing. *Archives of General Psychiatry, 62*, 1377–1384.

King, I. M. (1981). *A theory for nursing: Systems, concepts, process.* New York: John Wiley & Sons.

Knaus, W. A., Draper, E. A., Wagner, D. P., & Zimmerman, J. E. (1986). An evaluation of outcome from intensive care in major medical centers. *Annals of Internal Medicine, 104*, 410–418.

Lang, N. M. (1976). Issues in quality assurance in nursing. *Issues in Evaluation Research* [ANA Publication, ANA Publ. No. G-124], 45–56.

Lohr, K. N. (Ed.), and the Committee to Design a Strategy for Quality Review and Assurance in Medicare. (1990). *Medicare: A strategy for quality assurance.* Washington, DC: Institute of Medicine, National Academy of Sciences, National Academy Press.

Mashek, D. J., & Aron, A. (2004). *Handbook of closeness and intimacy.* Philadelphia, PA: Lawrence Erlbaum.

Meyer, B., & Bishop, D. S. (2007). Florence Nightingale: Nineteenth century apostle of quality. *Journal of Management History, 13*(3), 240–253.

Mitchell, P., Ferketich, S., & Jennings, B. M. (1998). American Academy of Nursing Expert Panel on Quality Health Care—Quality Health Outcomes Model. *Journal of Nursing Scholarship, 30*(1), 43–46.

National Center for Complementary and Alternative Medicine. (2007). Retrieved December 4, 2007, from http://nccam.nih.gov/health/backgrounds/mindbody.htm

Naylor, M. (2003). Nursing intervention research and quality of care: Influencing the future of healthcare. *Nursing Research, 52*(6), 380–385.

Nightingale, F. (1859). *Notes on nursing: What it is and what it is not.* Philadelphia, PA: J. B. Lippincott.

Orem, D. (2001). *Nursing concepts of practice* (6th ed.). Wilkes Barre, PA: CV Mosby.

Peplau, H. E. (1988). *Interpersonal relations in nursing.* New York: Springer Publishing.

Rippentrop, E. A., Altmaier, E. M., Chen, J. J., Found, E. M., & Keffala, V. J. (2005). The relationship between religion/spirituality and physical health, mental health, and pain in a chronic pain population. *Pain, 116*(3), 311–321.

Rogers, C. (1961). On becoming a person: A therapist's view of psychotherapy. *Archives of General Psychiatry, 62*, 1377–1384.

Roy, C. (1980). The Roy Adaptation Model. In J. P. Riehl & C. Roy (Eds.), *Conceptual models for nursing practice* (2nd ed., pp. 179–188). New York: Appleton-Century-Crofts.

Safran, D. G., Miller, W., & Beckman, H. (2006). Organizational dimensions of relationship-centered care: Theory, evidence, and practice. *Journal of General Internal Medicine, 21*(S1), S9–S15.

Stacey, R. (2001). *Complex response process in organizations: Learning and knowledge creation.* London: Routledge.

Suchman, A. S. (2006). A new theoretical foundation for relationship-centered care complex responsive processes of relating. *Journal of General Internal Medicine, 21*(S1), S40–S44.

Thomas, E. J., Sherwood, G., & Helmreich, R. L. (2003). Lessons from aviation: Teamwork to improve patient safety. *Nursing Economics, 21*(5), 241–243.

Travelbee, J. (1966). *Interpersonal aspects of nursing.* Philadelphia, PA: FA Davis.

Tresolini, C. P., & The Pew-Fetzer Task Force. (1994). *Health professions education and relationship-centered care.* San Francisco, CA: Pew Health Professions Commission.

Watson, J. (1979). *Nursing: The philosophy and science of caring.* Boston: Little, Brown and Company.

Watson, J. (1985). *Nursing: Human science and human care.* Norwalk, CT: Appleton-Century-Crofts.

Williams, R. L. (1994). *Essentials of total quality management.* New York: Amacom.

Relationship-Centered Caring

3 Caring for Self

The key to humanity's future lies in the productive linkage of the mind, body and spirit.

—John E. Fetzer

Keywords: self, balance, interaction, self-caring

THE PROMISING SELF

As psychossocioculturalspiritual beings, humans exist in relationship to others and their environment and, to a larger extent, the universe. Humans also exist as individuals, separate from other people, with unique characteristics. Philosophically, human beings are differentiated from other forms of life by features such as consciousness, the ability to reason and move autonomously, and the capacity to use language. From most formal religious perspectives, such uniqueness confers respect, dignity, and value for human life.

Through life experiences and normal growth processes, humans develop throughout the lifespan biologically, cognitively (Piaget, 1972, 1990), psychologically (Buhler, 1972; Buhler & Marschak, 1967; Erikson, 1964, 1968; Gould, 1978; Havighurst, 1953; Jung, 1933; Levinson, 1966; Levinson, Darrow, & Klein, 1978; Sheehy, 1976), morally (Kohlberg,

1986), and some would say spiritually, all influenced by specific socio-cultural dimensions, such as gender, race, and societal status. This complex blend of unique life forces influences each other and eventually the *whole* person (Clark & Caffarella, 1999). Such an integrated perspective of human development, which is increasingly becoming the dominant worldview, is considered too complicated to understand from just one perspective.

Transpersonal psychology grew out of the humanistic movement and adds a spiritual or "higher consciousness" dimension to adult development and focuses on the unity and connectiveness of all things. It views humans as capable of cognitive and psychological growth through all phases of life, which has implications for learning, optimum health, and positive relationships. A key to such human growth is self-awareness or clarity about one's relationship to the environment, other people, and perceptions of reality. This awareness of both subjective and objective phenomena in life is not static; rather, it occurs on a continuum from being fully awake and aware of oneself to being asleep or unaware (Schlitz, Vieten, & Amorok, 2007).

Subjective or internally focused self-awareness grounds the self to see with clarity how life experiences shape thoughts and behaviors. Concepts such as the perception of the physical body or body image, self-concept, agency (one's capacity to act), or social identity are understood and refined as self-awareness or consciousness is heightened. Such a view of humans suggests a depth of understanding is possible that may empower one to advance his/her full potential, have meaningful relationships, and achieve some form of contentment or peace.

Unfortunately, as humans go about relating, working, and caring for each other, the self is often forgotten or lost along the way. Disappointments, insecurities, losses, physical ailments, and the everyday fast-paced demands of life build up over time leaving many stressed and exhausted. In such a state, individuals tend to function more on "automatic pilot" where activities become habitual or mechanistic. To make matters worse, learned ways of knowing (externally derived) such as formal education and religious training may limit or focus the view of oneself. In this restricted view of the world, individuals tend to be more reactive, feel separated or disjointed, and function under an individualistic or misplaced view of the world. Nurses, in particular, tend to "get used to the pressure and lose sight of just how much they have to deal with" (Rainham, 1994, p. 6); in fact, many nurses are proud of their multitasking abilities! But balancing highly acute patient needs, poor staffing, the physical demands of nurse work, and making life and death decisions according to the latest evidence along with family responsibilities, traffic, and 24/7 information overload leaves many nurses feeling drained and worn out. Such emotions, without awareness of them, begin to grow into general dissatisfaction and even physical symptoms. Balancing internal authentic awareness of self along with external worldly views may strengthen one such that an integrated, more resilient and healthy self is more available (see Figure 3.1).

Exciting new empirical evidence is beginning to emerge that demonstrates the connections between emotions and physiological processes. The mind–body intelligence (MBI) approach recognizes individuals as both emotional and physiological beings functioning within families, social groups (including work groups), and communities (Adelman, 2006).

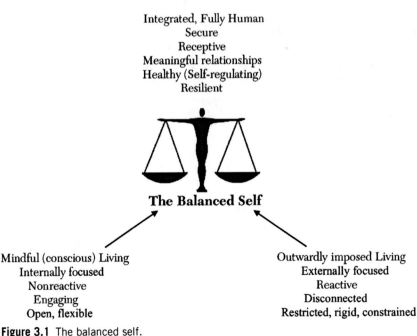

Integrated, Fully Human
Secure
Receptive
Meaningful relationships
Healthy (Self-regulating)
Resilient

The Balanced Self

Mindful (conscious) Living
Internally focused
Nonreactive
Engaging
Open, flexible

Outwardly imposed Living
Externally focused
Reactive
Disconnected
Restricted, rigid, constrained

Figure 3.1 The balanced self.

Under the rubric of self-awareness, using special meditation, mindfulness, prayer, the arts, and relaxation techniques, research is beginning to demonstrate a link between MBI and decreased stress, increased quality of life, and self-compassion (Shapiro, Astin, Bishop, & Cordova, 2005). Regularly practicing these activities helps an individual come to understand his/her strengths and weaknesses; this appreciation helps one to recognize the early signs of unconscious, preoccupied, or mindless living. Paying attention to oneself is important for effective authentic interaction, health (Davidson et al., 2003), and the capacity to care for others (Siegel, 2007).

INTERACTING WITH THE SELF

Professional nurses interact and relate to others with ease; yet, nurses have not traditionally been taught how to do this for themselves. In an earlier concept analysis of the term *relating*, Lamb (1998) refers to establishing bonds and meaningful interaction as an explanation. She lists characteristics such as acceptance, valuing, empathetic understanding, sensitivity, and trust as necessary to effective relating. Finally, she describes learning to relate as an ongoing process that requires initiative and choice.

Permitting oneself to slow down enough to actually focus on one's inner thoughts and feelings allows one to access his/her phenomenal field or subjective reality. Once accessed, this attention to self helps one see his/her situation clearly. In turn, such actions may help nurses appreciate and honor the work they do.

In the work environment, regular efforts to increase conscious awareness may help professional nurses focus more readily on the important aspects of nurse work, such as holistically assessing patients' needs, making clinical judgments, and using best evidence, versus mindless tasking. Short pauses between patient rooms, taking brief time-outs to sit and ponder, and using routine tasks such as handwashing, charting, or walking from room to room as opportunities to feel one's body and emotions may in fact be therapeutic to both the patient and the nurse.

Reflective awareness by soliciting simple feedback from patients or coworkers is a more advanced and objective form of raising awareness. In an unsure moment, asking patients "How did I do?" is most appropriate because it provides information from the most reliable source. Validating intuitive thoughts or objective findings about patients with other nurses or health care providers helps nurses learn to trust themselves and builds confidence. Most nurses have been taught "to do," to help patients solve problems, to teach, and to provide answers. In fact, task or activity dominance (being observed as busy) is considered proper behavior for nurses. Yet, patients enter the health care system with a wealth of knowledge about their illnesses and their own ways of solving problems. Sometimes, just "being there" fully present in the moment allows patients the opportunity to use their own knowledge and skills while the nurse provides guidance and support. All of these more mindful activities require openness to new ideas, flexibility, and tolerance on the part of the nurse. If taught to honor themselves early on, nurses may come to view such behaviors as less threatening.

Reflective analysis is a higher form of interacting with self in which the expression of thoughts and feelings is actually written down, spoken into a recorder, or videotaped and then analyzed according to some format. Such analysis requires taking the time to ponder thought processes (such as what one is really thinking) and actions (such as why one acted a certain way or how one arrived at a decision). Approaching this self-introspection with openness and curiosity (to both positive and negative aspects of the self) uncovers the hidden meanings and learning opportunities that occurred during clinical work and helps integrate them into future practice. This form of interacting with the self is regularly used in nursing education but is often discarded upon graduation.

PRACTICING SELF-CARING

As shown through theory and recent research, taking time to gain insight into emotions, thoughts, bodily sensations, and other feelings contributes to well-being and may be a necessary antecedent to caring for others. Professional nurses need to acknowledge and allow themselves to feel the meanings associated with nurse work, including suffering. As Foster (2004) explains, "When nurses fail at their own healthcare, it shows in workplace relationships, sick days, burnout, and turnover" (p. 112).

Making time for true relaxation—not just time off from work—but authentic quiet time by oneself is essential. Nursing is so people-oriented and other-focused that time alone is often not seen as valuable. Yet, alone-time can become a practice that enhances self-caring.

In fact, in the classic *Solitude* (1988), Anthony Storr states, "The capacity to be alone . . . becomes linked with self-discovery and self-actualization; with becoming aware of one's deepest needs, feelings, and impulses" (p. 21). In the nursing culture of self-sacrifice and adrenalin-induced nervous energy, creating balance through regular private time is self-therapeutic. For example, a few minutes alone practicing deep breathing or taking a leisurely walk by oneself can promote insight and help one reframe a situation or experience harmony and a sense of peace. In the work situation, during particularly busy times, just taking a minute or two to consciously breathe or count is a renewing activity that may in fact help nurses connect more or refocus on the important meaning of their work.

Likewise, committing to private time each day is a requisite for quality nursing care. Just like physical exercise, obligating oneself to quiet time requires altering of daily habits. Waking up 15 minutes early or creating an evening ritual of quiet time during which one practices meditation, contemplative prayer, or just sitting quietly with oneself is essential to nurses' well-being. These kinds of experiences help one become attuned to the larger whole, allowing connections to surface that might otherwise remain buried.

The key word here is *practice;* a verb, practice requires *action*. Mindfulness practices require several essential elements (Schlitz et al., 2007). First is *intention* or making the choice to stay open and aware. Second is *directing attention inward;* in other words being present to the self. Third, committing to a more conscious way of living requires *repetition*.

Repeating components of a mindfulness practice reinforces the habit. Finally, *guidance* in the form of both external learning and/or accessing internal wisdom can increase the value of mindfulness practices.

Several methods are available to practice mindful awareness. Deep relaxation and meditation practices, yoga and tai chi, contemplative prayer, walking, rehearsing a song, even service itself, when acted in a conscious manner, can be transpersonal experiences. The key to such practices are the four essential elements (Schlitz et al., 2007). In the personal practice of deep relaxation, for example, making the commitment (intent) to devote the necessary time as well as focused attention to breathing or other bodily functions, repeating the practice in the same way and at the same time each day, and reading about or taking a class on relaxation techniques are all reinforcers that enable the practice to bring clarity to the self. Expression of oneself through artistic or creative pursuits, such as music, painting, sewing, quilting, gardening, woodworking, or noncompetitive sports, when consciously pursued, can be awareness-raising. These activities keep us "in the moment" and, although considered recreation, with the right intent, attention, repetition, and guidance, they can provide the same accessibility to the self as more traditional practices (Schlitz et al., 2007). In the case of music, there is some evidence that it may even be physically and emotionally therapeutic (Sachs, 2007).

Another way to access the inner self is to spend time in nature. Professional nurses are most often working in drab, enclosed environments with artificial lighting and temperature controls. Often, there are no windows or opportunities to even see the outside surroundings. Being in the natural environment and using the experience to appreciate its mystery provide a reflective time to ponder about the interconnectedness of the universe. In this way, one can learn to quiet the self and see the sacred in everyday life. Taking a walk around the building at lunchtime or sitting near a window while eating in the cafeteria may help assist nurses during their working hours.

Reflective awareness, a form of self-observation, allows an individual to examine oneself through the eyes of another. Using ordinary circumstances, this form of practicing self-caring involves soliciting feedback about one's actions or behaviors from those who were involved in the same experience but from a different perspective. For example, during the personal experience of a difficult parent–adolescent interaction, the parent might ask for feedback from the child about the quality of the interaction. Questions such as how could we have reached a conclusion sooner? or what did I do that particularly annoyed you? yield new perspectives that the parent can integrate into future interactions.

In the practice setting, a nurse might ask another nurse to comment on his/her interactions with a family member. Questions such as what did you see me do that was helpful to this family? or what nonverbal behaviors did you observe in the interaction? help the nurse see his/herself through the lens of the recipient of care. This perspective, when listened to and acted upon, can be a powerful tool for learning about the self and validating or changing behaviors.

Reflective analysis is a more formal practice that involves thinking about a situation, describing it through narrative writing, evaluating it, and, through the process, integrating what one has learned into future professional practice. Regular reflective analysis either as a group or individually helps nurses understand themselves, see patterns, build confidence, change behavior, and ultimately become more fully human (Lauterbach & Becker, 1996). An example of reflective analysis occurred during a class on nurse–patient interactions (The Catholic University of America, 2006). The instructor asked the RN students to think of a time when they felt they had delivered *professional* nursing care and felt good about it. The students were directed to describe what they did and how they felt about it, assess why they felt good, and then summarize what they had learned from the situation that could inform their practice. Some excerpts from their responses are:

> The patient relayed to me that she was told the night before to use the diaper and that was very humiliating . . . so I made a deal with her that I would come in every hour to check if she wanted to use the commode, which I made sure I did . . . I was glad and proud of myself for taking care of such a small detail and how much that changed my day and the relationship with that patient.

> I saw that by spending those few extra minutes talking and listening, I was able to have a less stressful day and the patient was not pressed to seek my attention. I felt like the beginning of some healing may have taken place; that I was really nursing.

On my way home from work I ran through my day in my head. I zoomed in on my interaction with Mrs. P. I shouldn't have felt so annoyed with her I thought. But then I said to myself, "V, you are human. You get annoyed with your children but that does not mean you don't love them or care. Don't be so hard on yourself—when I last checked you were still human!" Taking time out and regrouping is important in order to provide emotional stability.

I was assigned to a young breast cancer patient (32 yrs old) who refused chemo. I had a similar experience and used this to care for her. My approach was to talk to the patient about the benefits of chemo, radiation and follow up. I gave her hope and encouraged her to follow up on the doctor's recommendations . . . I referred her to support groups. The patient eventually asked the doctor for treatment . . . I felt very pleased that I had made a difference in somebody's life—maybe even saved it. The patient thanked me for being there to listen to her concerns and guiding her during this critical time.

They told me his diaper needed to be changed. He had underwear over the diaper so I removed it, cleaned, and changed him and did not replace the underwear. His relatives then re-entered the room and I explained that, since he was having loose stools and we will be changing him often, I left the underwear off. They asked me to please put it on because he "wants to die with his underwear on." I followed their wishes and changed him four additional times—each time replacing his underwear. When I came to work the next day, I learned he had passed away early that morning. The news was expected. I thought to myself how important it was that I honored his wishes and he died in dignity.

Interestingly, these excerpts were elicited from a question related to *professional* nursing care. Each of them occurred in a situation where there was interaction between the patient and nurse, and the respondents felt good about it. It appears that the RNs in this class felt they had performed *professionally* when the dominant activity of the nurse was caring relationships with patients and families!

Another example of reflective analysis occurred in an organization that had implemented a caring professional practice model during the preceding year. During the annual evaluation process, the nurses were asked to write out how their practice had changed since the adoption of the model, and secondly, they were asked to describe an experience they had with the model that had informed their practice. In general, the responses reflected that the nurses sensed that more direct time spent with patients and families allowed them to establish open, trusting communication, provide reassurance and advocate for patients, and be more "in tune" to their patients' comfort needs, and it motivated their practice. Some specific responses included:

> The fact that I take the time to know the patient not only as patient but as a Mom/Dad, a professional, has given me a different perspective in the way I view/treat the patient. I have slowed down.

> I made a point to compliment the ED nurse for good work. I also called and left a message with her manager about this good work . . . It felt good to give some positive reinforcement.

> I had a patient who was combative, noncommunicative and with dementia. He was challenging to handle but I imagined that if he were my father, I would want him treated with care.

> Now I feel I am really practicing nursing—I started to think more about my responsibility and accountability.

> I had 3 patients—one needing pain meds q 2 hrs and the other 2 needing pain med q 3 hrs. I started becoming agitated in report telling the charge nurse this was an unfair assignment. But then I thought to myself, "you can have a bad day or you can refocus and re-center yourself."

These written reflections were brought to the annual evaluation process and discussed together with the nurse manager. The discussions allowed both the nurse managers and the staff nurses to think aloud about the new model, use the results of the analysis to revise practice, and, in some cases, design new educational activities as well as set up the conditions for promotion.

Of course, taking care of the body through regular exercise and healthy eating are self-caring acts that many nurses forget to do for themselves as they take care of others. Yet, caring for the physical body is crucial to quality nursing practice. And, the particularly serious nature of health care often diminishes opportunities to see some of the lighter sides of human nature. The use of humor, particularly in the workplace, can be a source of joy even in the most difficult of circumstances (Wooten, 1996). Establishing a support network or taking classes that reinforce and help perfect awareness practices enhances their performance. Monitoring oneself during working hours by regularly observing one's behavior and asking, "Am I stressed or at ease?" or "Am I busy doing or am I present to myself, my co-workers and my patients?" keeps one alert and in the moment. Regular reminders to practice mindfulness, such as keeping relaxation CDs in the car and pictures or other symbols in the workplace, may assist nurses to practice mindfulness daily.

Improving awareness by allowing oneself to feel physical as well as emotional sensations, reflecting on them slowly, making meaning of them, and using this introspection to relate to others in a continual pattern of action and inaction keeps one balanced and more "in tune" to the world's energy. The regular performance of personal and professional self-caring practices sets up the conditions for self-knowing, a prerequisite for helping others.

KNOWING THE SELF

As humans have the capacity to continuously learn and grow, it follows that practicing mindfulness both personally and professionally may have the potential to positively influence lives—both our own and those we care for. According to Siegel (2007), personal mindfulness practices (such as meditation, deep relaxation, prayer, etc.) lead to self-wisdom and even decreased negative states such as depression and anger (Sephton et al., 2007). Such practices also lead to improved positive states such as increased compassion for self. In other words, personal mindfulness practices create the possibility for well-being. In addition, empirical evidence is beginning to emerge that actually shows structural differences in brain tissue (Baer, Smith, Hoskins, Krietemeyer, & Toney, 2006), connections between mindfulness practices and increased brain tissue (Lazar et al., 2005), increased perception of time (Tse, 2005), and decreased psychological suffering in those who regularly practice mindfulness. Although this research is preliminary, it is compelling that some persons who regularly practice conscious awareness have different or additional areas of brain tissue and less distress in their lives.

In Figure 3.2, both personal and empirical ways of knowing are presented. Siegel (2007) contends that with practice and training we can learn to be mindful. If this is so, it is reasonable to speculate that individuals can learn how to recognize and adjust their emotions to decrease negative states and increase positive states (i.e., to self-advance). In a qualitative study of intractable conflict, subjects were taught mindfulness approaches that promoted resolution through growing awareness, accepting reality, regaining equilibrium, and cognitively and emotionally gaining internal control. Such an approach allowed the participants to

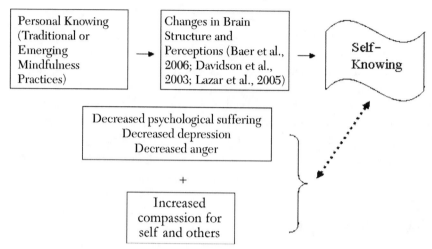

Figure 3.2 Self-knowing.

reframe the situation, make decisions, and resolve interpersonal conflict (Horton-Deutsch & Horton, 2003). Over time, one might ask, can this activity actually remodel brain tissue?

If the emerging evidence is correct, knowing the self may lead to knowing the other in a more caring manner. Knowing the self includes valuing the self and the profession and regularly examining personal and professional experiences to illuminate their essential aspects and learn from them. Valuing the self includes appreciating the internal meanings (along with the externally imposed meanings) of our experiences in order to change perceptions, build confidence, and create positive workplaces. Just as nurses do with patients, creating and implementing a plan for self-caring is an essential aspect for attaining health.

SUMMARY

The focus of this chapter centered on the self—its promising nature and the internal and external ways of knowing it. Evidence of the link between the mind and some physiologic changes was presented. A description of three ways of raising consciousness—increasing awareness during everyday activities, reflective awareness through feedback from others, and the more formal reflective analysis format—was explained. Examples of applications pertinent to busy nurses, such as silent time alone, specific practices, creative arts, physical exercise and nutrition, and soliciting feedback from others, were highlighted. Two examples of reflective analysis provide insight to professional nursing practice. Knowing and valuing the self—both personally and empirically—was introduced as a prerequisite for caring interactions.

CALLS TO ACTION

Slowing down enough to contact one's inner world—thoughts, desires, feelings—permits one to gain access to his/her own reality. Linking to this valuable resource of self helps nurses remember what they already know—the powerful nature of their work. **Recognize** nursing's power.

Balancing external and internal energy requires regularly disengaging oneself from the nursing culture of tension, multitasking, and acquiescence to one of quiet aloneness—such action is renewing. **Sit** in silent reflection for 15 minutes this week.

Reflective Questions/Applications for Students

1. Explain the term *consciousness.*
2. Explain how you might use reflective awareness with a coworker; your husband/wife; a patient.
3. Explain the three forms of self-awareness highlighted in this chapter.
4. Think of a nurse who exemplifies caring. Describe his/her characteristics. What can you learn from this person?
5. Using a developmental psychology framework, discuss how humans continue to grow, learn, and evolve throughout the lifespan.
6. HOW WELL DO YOU KNOW YOURSELF? (answer the following questions and then sit in silence for 15 minutes reflecting on the answers).

   I am proud of _____
   I would like to _____

I have learned that _____
I regret _____
I am annoyed about _____
I am frightened by _____
I am disgusted by _____
I wonder about _____
I enjoy _____
I need _____
I hope _____
I want _____

7. Develop a plan for self-caring. Specifically describe the aware-
    ness practice/s you use now or will choose to access your au-
    thentic self. Include details about how you will commit to the
    practice, how you will structure your attention, what repetitive
    components you will use, and the external guidance you will
    seek to perfect the practice.
8. Describe a nursing situation in which you think you did not
    perform up to your *professional* potential. What happened?
    How did you react? What challenges did you face? What con-
    clusions did you draw about your strengths and opportunities
    for growth from the situation? What changes, if any, do you
    plan to make to improve your practice?
9. Design a Web-based reflective analysis process that can be reg-
    ularly used by nurses in your workplace. Write a procedure for
    accessing, maintaining confidentiality, and using the practice.
10. Make a network of support diagram. Place yourself in the cen-
    ter. Then drawing out from the center, depict all those people,
    places, activities, or environments from which you experience
    support. Under each of these, list the characteristics that make
    this resource supportive.

Reflective Questions/Applications for Educators

11. What would you do differently in clinical courses to help stu-
    dents center themselves?
12. How would you encourage students to ask for feedback on
    their performance?
13. Develop a plan for self-caring. Specifically describe the aware-
    ness practice/s you use now or will choose to access your au-
    thentic self. Include details about how you will commit to the

practice, how you will structure your attention, what repetitive components you will use, and the external guidance you will seek to perfect the practice.

Reflective Questions/Applications for Nurse Leaders

14. What can you do or what reminders can you create in your work environment to prompt nurses to focus their awareness on the important work they do?

15. Develop a plan for self-caring. Specifically describe the awareness practice/s you use now or will choose to access your authentic self. Include details about how you will commit to the practice, how you will structure your attention, what repetitive components you will use, and the external guidance you will seek to perfect the practice.

REFERENCES

Adelman, E. M. (2006). Mind-body intelligence: A new perspective integrating Eastern and Western healing traditions. *Holistic Nursing Practice, 20*(3), 147–151.

Baer, R. A., Smith, G. T., Hoskins, J., Krietemeyer, J., & Toney, L. (2006). Using self-report assessment methods to explore facets of mindfulness. *Assessment, 13*(1), 27–45.

Buhler, C., & Allen, M. (1972). *Introduction to humanistic psychology.* Monterey, CA: Brooks/Cole Publishing Co.

Buhler, C., & Marschak, M. (1967). Basic tendencies of human life. In C. Buhler & F. Massarik (Eds.), *The course of human life.* New York: Springer Publishing.

The Catholic University of America. (2006). *Nursing 567: Relationship-centered caring.* Spring.

Clark, M. C., & Caffarella, R. S. (1999). An update on adult development: New ways of thinking about the life course. *New directions for adult and continuing education.* San Francisco, CA: Jossey-Bass.

Davidson, R. J., Kabat-Zinn, J., Schumacher, J., Rosenkranz, M., Muller, D., Santorelli, S. F., et al. (2003). Alterations in brain and immune function produced by mindfulness meditation. *Psychosomatic Medicine, 65*(4), 564–570.

Erikson, E. H. (1964). *Insight and responsibility.* New York: Norton.

Erikson, E. H. (1968). *Identity: Youth and crisis.* New York: Norton.

Foster, R. (2004). Self-care: Why is it so hard? *Journal of Specialists in Pediatric Nursing, 9*(4), 111–112.

Gould, R. (1978). *Transformations: Growth and change in adult life.* New York: Simon & Schuster.

Havighurst, R. (1953). *Human development and education.* New York: McKay.

Horton-Deutsch, S. L., & Horton, J. M. (2003). Mindfulness: Overcoming intractable conflict. *Archives of Psychiatric Nursing, 17*(4), 186–193.

Jung, C. (1933). *Modern man in search of a soul.* New York: Harcourt, Brace & Co.

Kohlberg, L. (1986). *The philosophy of moral development.* San Francisco, CA: Harper and Row.

Lamb, M. A. (1998). Concept analysis of relating: A human response. *International Journal of Nursing Terminology and Classification, 9*(1), 15–21.

Lauterbach, S. S., & Becker, P. H. (1996). Caring for self: Becoming a self-reflective nurse. *Holistic Nursing Practice, 10*(2), 57–68.

Lazar, S. W., Kerr, C. E., Wasserman, R. H., Gray, J. R., Greve, D., Treadway, M. T., et al. (2005). Meditation experience is associated with increased cortical thickness. *Neuroreport, 16,* 1893–1897.

Levinson, D. J. (1966). *Seasons of a woman's life.* New York: Alfred A. Knopf.

Levinson, D. J., with Darrow, C. N., & Klein, E. B. (1978). *Seasons of a man's life.* New York: Random House.

Piaget, J. (1972). *The psychology of the child.* New York: Basic Books.

Piaget, J. (1990). *The child's conception of the world.* New York: Littlefield Adams.

Rainham, D. C. (1994). *The stress of nursing: Meeting the challenge.* Waterloo, MI: Optimum Health Resources.

Sachs, O. (2007). *Musicophilia: Tales of music and the brain.* New York: Alfred A. Knopf.

Schlitz, M. M., Vieten, C., & Amorok, T. (2007). *Living deeply: The art and science of transformation in everyday life.* Oakland, CA: New Harbinger Publications, Inc.

Sephton, S. E., Salmon, P., Weissbecker, I., Ulmer, C., Floyd, A., Hoover, K., et al. (2007). Mindfulness meditation alleviates depressive symptoms in women with fibromyalgia: Results of a randomized clinical trial. *Arthritis Care and Research, 57*(1), 77–85.

Shapiro, S. L., Astin, J. A., Bishop, S., & Cordova, M. (2005). Mindfulness-based stress reduction for health care professionals: Results from a randomized trial. *International Journal of Stress Management, 12,* 164–176.

Sheehy, G. (1976). *Passages: Predictable crises of adult life.* New York: E. P. Dutton.

Siegel, D. J. (2007). *The mindful brain.* New York: W.W. Norton & Company.

Storr, A. (1988). *Solitude.* New York: Free Press.

Tse, P. U. (2005). Voluntary attention modulates the brightness of overlapping transparent surfaces. *Vision Research, 45*(9), 1095–1098.

Wooten, P. (1996). Laughter as therapy for patient and caregiver. In J. Hodgkin, G. Connors, & C. Bell (Eds.), *Pulmonary rehabilitation.* Philadelphia, PA: Lippincott.

4 Caring for Patients and Families

I am a part of all that I have seen.

—Alfred Lord Tennyson

Keywords: illness, intention, caring factors

THE IMPACT OF ILLNESS ON PATIENTS AND FAMILIES

As complex beings that are constantly changing and relating, humans have objective (physical), subjective (emotional, spiritual), social (family and role functions), and cultural characteristics. During an illness these characteristics are affected, and the results are profound. First, there is the reaction to and necessary adjustment to the illness itself. Illness represents a fundamental threat to one's basic sense of wholeness. Persons may form certain meanings about their illnesses based on the knowledge they have about their own body, what they have heard or read about others in similar situations, individual psychological significances, and societal/cultural points of view. Physiological changes can create feelings of discomfort, vulnerability, and dependence that generate loss of self-confidence and create uncertainty. Ambitions or plans must be suspended, and communication patterns change. Fulfilling one's role as parent, grandparent, spouse, worker, or friend is often disrupted, and the psychological impact of being ill presents threats to one's sense of wholeness. Oftentimes, persons experience shock, anger, or fear as the initial emotional response to a diagnosis or need for care from others. Over time, these emotions may change and can be viewed on a continuum from courageous acceptance on the one hand to specific self-destructive behaviors that can lead to personal and family turmoil on the other hand.

Consider older adults who are hospitalized. This vulnerable group is diverse with many comorbidities, multiple medication and treatment regimens, complex discharge needs, and health insurance problems (Center for Disease Control and Prevention, 2003). In addition, hospitalization for older adults can represent the beginning of functional decline and increased dependence (Chang et al., 2003). Once admitted, older adults must take on the dependent role of patient and conform to the disjointed health care system including the fast-paced, highly technological environment (Institute of Medicine, 2001). Consequently, hospitalized older adults may experience stress and sleeplessness (Topf & Thompson, 2001), feel insecure and devalued (Williams & Iruita, 2004), report dissatisfaction with care, are particularly at risk for adverse outcomes (CDC, 2004), experience functional decline (Sager & Rudberg, 1998), and often are discharged without the requisite knowledge and skills to care for themselves (Williams, 2004). These disparities are profound and growing, often intensified by cultural insensitivities. Chopra (2004) reminds us that, once hospitalized, "patients are helpless under the authority of doctors and nurses; they are dehumanized by the cold mechanistic routine, isolated from everyday society, made more or less anonymous as one 'case' among thousands" (p. 130).

Within the family, changes in spousal relationships frequently take place as a result of an illness. Often, a shift in balance among members of a family leaves children, in particular, frightened or upset, regardless of the parent's age. Some members miss work or give up leisure activities to care for a loved one. Finally, how individual family members cope with the illness varies; some need open discussion, while others require time alone. All of these changes are trumped by the direct and opportunity costs associated with illness. With the rise in the older population and associated chronic disease, demands on family members will continue. Coping with these demands places enormous burdens on family members' emotional, social, and financial well-being.

As patients and their families present to the health care system for needed care, they are compromised based on their illnesses, but they are also compromised based on the threats to their sense of personal and societal meaning. Hospitalization unintentionally contributes to these threats by the incessant stream of complete strangers who invade patients' personal space, the labeling of patients according to diagnoses, the rules patients have to follow, and the impersonal communication patients receive. Thus, central to providing high-quality care is the ability of health care providers to "experience the other person's private world and feelings and to communicate to the other person some significant degree of that understanding" (Watson, 1979, p. 28). Such behavior on the part of the nurse requires the *intention* to care.

CARING INTENTION

Caring is an intentional process that requires self-awareness, choice, specific knowledge and skills, and time (Duffy & Hoskins, 2003) (see Figure 4.1).

The word *intentional* is important because it forms the basis for choosing behavior. Husserl (1980) identified intention as a phenomenological trait that characterizes a mental state or experience as being "directed toward something." Fishbein and Ajzen (1975) defined intention

- Knowledge   Caring Factors
  Four required relationships (self, patients and families, health team, community)

- Skills   behaviors, competencies

- Intention   attitudes, beliefs ⟶ choice

- Time   primary focus on relationships
  integration of "being" and "doing"

Figure 4.1 Requirements for caring professional practice.

as involving four elements: the behavior, the target object, the situation, and the time the behavior is being performed. On the basis of their empirical studies, Fishbein and Ajzen proposed that the formation of a given intention depends on prior development of a particular attitude together with a person's subjective beliefs. *Attitude* consists of beliefs about the consequences of performing the behavior and the person's evaluation of these consequences. The *subjective* piece is related to an individual's perceptions of how others would view them if they performed the behavior. In simple terms, intention is the resolve to act based on the combination of attitude toward the behavior and subjective norms. *Caring intention,* then, influences the choice to care (for a particular person in a particular place and time). Making a conscious (fully aware) choice to be caring is a consequence of caring intention.

Perugini and Bagozzi (2004) differentiated intention from desire through two studies. They found that desires are more abstract, less feasible, and less connected to action, whereas intention is related to action and behavior. However, these analyses did point to the fact that desire is an important predictor of intention.

In nursing terms, one may desire to spend time with patients, but the commitment to it may vacillate, and the intention (attitude and beliefs about spending time) and perhaps the resultant behavior may not occur. Caring intention relates to a nurse's attitude and experiential meanings of caring actions. Such a definition implies one would *know* or be conscious of the benefits of caring prior to its initiation; using this awareness, the nurse directs his/her attention toward the patient and displays the intention through purposeful behavior.

Caring intention is behaviorally oriented and is not to be confused with the term *intentionality.* Intentionality refers to a state of being or one's whole frame of reference at a point in time. It signifies a deep or a grounding dimension that sets the stage for *how* one directs his/her thoughts. Watson (1999) spoke to intentionality (a verb) as a higher form of consciousness that allows one to deliberately see alternatives and influence outcomes.

Developing caring attitudes and meanings occurs through one's lived experiences of caring as well as through learning human caring acts by studying, self-reflecting, and observing members of one's profession. These experiences and external sources combined with the more internal understanding of oneself together enhance caring capacity. As one becomes more aware, purposeful, and centered, caring intention emerges in relationships; associated behaviors become more authentic, even reverent. Nursing's caring intention is apparent when behavior is positively directed toward the patient/family or other health team members using caring factors to initiate, cultivate, and sustain relationships.

CARING FACTORS

Several health care providers have documented certain factors as necessary for therapeutic relationships (Rogers, 1961; Yalom, 1975). Watson (1979, 1985) identified 10 factors necessary for human caring in the nurse–patient relationship. She identified the first 3—altruism, faith-hope, and sensitivity to self and others—as foundational. Recently, these factors have been revised and are now labeled Clinical Carative Processes (Watson, 2006). To empirically validate these dimensions, Duffy, Hoskins, and Seifert (2007) completed an exploratory factor analysis of the concept *caring*. They found 8 factors, each independently explaining caring. Although limited by the convenient sample, this study provides preliminary empirical support for several factors that comprise caring.

Mutual problem solving emerged as the largest factor and includes nursing behaviors that help patients and families understand how to confront, learn, and think about their health and illness. Using this knowledge, both parties decide together how to approach and solve problems in an acceptable manner to both. Behaviors such as providing information, reframing, helping patients learn, exploring alternative ways of dealing with health problems, brainstorming together, figuring out questions to ask, and checking with patients and families to validate what they know about their illnesses were deemed as important in this sample. Accepting feedback from patients and families and experimenting with different ways of doing things are also activities that communicate this factor. For example, chronic patients often enter a hospital for an episodic need and have established routines for caring for themselves. Listening to how patients care for themselves at home and adopting similar practices in the hospital can be comforting to the patient and more efficient for the nurse.

This factor implies that nurses are informed, are comfortable "in relationship," listen, use the patient–nurse relationship as the basis for teaching and learning, and are continuously learning and engaging patients and families in mutual discussions of their health problems.

Similar behaviors have been cited by others as important caring behaviors (Peplau, 1988; Swanson, 1991; Watson, 1979, 1985; Wolf, Zuelo, Goldberg, Crowthers, & Jacobson, 2006).

The second factor, *attentive reassurance,* refers to availability and hopeful outlook. "Patients in this sample viewed nurses as caring when they were accessible and optimistically able to look forward to the future (whatever that may be)" (Duffy et al., 2007, p. 240). Repeated confirmation of availability affects expectations of future availability; it assures patients and families that they can rely on the nurse, and a sense of security develops. Patients, despite their illnesses, wanted nurses who were confident and able to convey possibilities; to do this, nurses had to pay special attention to patients and families and encourage forward thinking.

> Paying attention to patients implies postponing action long enough to be authentically available—to notice, actively listen, and focus. Acting this way requires conscious effort on the part of the nurse to remove other thoughts from the mind in order to concentrate on the patient; such action provides patients and families with an anticipated future that is pleasurable. It is an uplifting feeling that may enhance the healing process.

Reassurance in this instance does not refer to the typical statement, "don't worry, everything will be alright." Such a statement may, in fact, not be true (in the case of one with a poor prognosis or another who faces a lifetime of chronic illness). But, more importantly, it is often said by the nurse to alleviate his/her own feelings about the situation (so he/she can move on) and may offer little support (and perhaps may be anxiety-provoking) to the patient. In fact, telling someone who is ill that "everything will be alright" often sets up a situation where the patient will stop expressing him/herself (because they intuitively know that this cannot be true). Sometimes just sitting with someone who is ill is reassuring; offering information about the safety of certain procedures, using gentle touch, or clarifying misperceptions are nursing behaviors that convey confidence and optimism. The appropriate use of humor is oftentimes considered reassuring because it lightens the perceived threat of illness. This caring factor actually has two components: attention and reassurance. Both are necessary ingredients for caring relationships.

Human respect, the third identified factor, refers to honoring the worth of humans by displaying behaviors such as unconditional acceptance, careful and kind handling of the human body, and recognition of rights and responsibilities. Most nursing theorists speak to respect for persons, and this factor is congruent with Watson's (1979, 1985) humanistic–altruistic value system, Boykin and Schoenhofer's (1993) unconditional acceptance, and Wolf and colleagues' (2006) showing respect dimensions of caring. This factor reminds nurses of the unique person behind the disease and the associated ethical principles that undergird nursing practice (American Nurses Association, 2001).

Regardless of age, physical or mental capacity, or social status, human persons who are ill are significant members of families, communities, and professions. Remembering this fact in the face of debilitating illness requires the nurse to appreciate the integrity of the patient (not just as a physical body), celebrating and talking about the patient's life when he/she is not ill, and working to ensure that the patient's honor is maintained. Especially in this global world where fellow humans sometimes look and act differently, realizing the interconnectedness and fundamental value of the human person is paramount. The simple act of calling a patient by his/her preferred name is a demonstration of respect. This factor conveys to a person that he or she matters.

Nurses were perceived as caring in this sample when they expressed an *encouraging manner.* This factor has an affective dimension because it refers to the demeanor or attitude of the nurse. Verbal as well as nonverbal messages convey this factor. For example, verbal messages of support spoken while body language suggests otherwise create incongruent messages that portray inauthenticity to the patient (see Table 4.1).

Table 4.1

ENCOURAGING VERSUS DISCOURAGING EXPRESSIONS

ENCOURAGING	DISCOURAGING
"I think you can do it."	"I'll do that."
"You're a hard worker."	"Be careful."
"I need your help with this."	"Don't forget to . . ."
"What can we do here?"	"Let's do this."

An encouraging approach suggests enthusiasm, support, positive commentary for effort, belief in the system, and empowerment. It assumes that persons are intrinsically motivated and have the ability to improve and grow. It allows room for patients and families to express their feelings, whether good or bad. It is the willingness to be open to all points of view. Even during bad experiences, an encouraging nurse who is poised and alert can point out some good aspects of a situation, however small. Patients in this sample expressed their desire for this attitude of encouragement to permeate nurses' way of behaving.

Appreciation of unique meanings is concerned with a patient's context or worldview. It refers to knowing what is important to patients including the distinctive sociocultural connections associated with their experiences.

Perceptions, thoughts, emotions, desires, bodily awareness, and actions have different meanings based on individuals' life circumstances. Nurses who use this caring factor avoid assumptions concerning patients and families; rather, they use those features that are important to them in the provision of care.

Appreciating unique meanings first involves discerning and then acknowledging in a positive way the subjective inner value attached to a situation, person, or event. Recognizing the significance of the patient's frame of reference implies a personal knowing that occurs over time in caring relationships. This factor is more an approach than a set of behaviors because it values the whole person of the patient together with the total experience of illness. Nurses who relate to patients and families in this manner often help them feel understood and capable.

Facilitating a *healing environment* has been considered a domain of nursing since Nightingale (1992). It refers to the setting where caring is taking place and is consistent with the views of human persons as holistic, complex beings in relationship; the surroundings, spaces, stressors (noise, lighting), and structures for maintaining patient privacy, safety, and control are aspects of this factor. In addition, a healing environment takes into account the organizational culture of a system including the vibrancy of the staff and management, workflow, access to spiritual resources, and features such as teamwork (or lack of it), norms of behavior (including the ability to ask questions and learn from mistakes in a nonpunitive manner), and resources. In fact, all of these factors are important to a culture of safety (Institute for Healthcare Improvement, 2008). Taking into account and acting when necessary to enhance the patient care environment is a major role of the nurse and one that may in fact be empirically tied to improved patient outcomes (Institute of Medicine, 2004).

Basic human needs are well known to nurses and include physical needs (air, food and fluids, elimination, sleep and rest), safety and security needs, social and relational needs, self-esteem needs, and self-actualization (Maslow, 1954, 1971). Recognizing the primacy of these needs during acute illness, including their comprehensiveness, is, however, many times not honored in the biomedically oriented health care environment. Often nurses concentrate on some of the physical needs because they are a symptom of the illness. But higher-order needs, such as social and self-esteem needs, are frequently forgotten. To complicate the situation, due to the increasing reliance on unlicensed assistive personnel, registered nurses often delegate meeting lower-order patient needs to others, or they aren't addressed at all. Yet patients in this sample viewed nurses as caring "when they made certain that their basic human needs were met" (Duffy et al., 2007, p. 242). When one perceives another as an integrated whole, the preciousness of the human person is not separate from one's illness, one's physical body, or one's thoughts and feelings. Caring for the physical body has traditionally been a time when professional nurses engage the patient, teach, assess, share dedicated time, and learn. Furthermore, the human body is a most intimate part of the self that deserves caring attention and respect.

When viewed in this manner, caring for the physical body is more than a bath, beyond mouth care, above feeding and ambulation. It is an opportunity for interaction that is personal and private. These human activities are common to us all and connect us to one another. They also provide evidence of the progression of an illness or the return to health. Do they not require the same consideration, knowledge, and skill as other nursing activities? If so, why are they relegated to nursing fundamentals texts or personnel without the requisite caring knowledge and skills?

Affiliation needs refer to persons' needs for belonging and membership in families or other social contexts. Many consider this factor a component of basic human needs, but it emerged as an independent factor, explaining 6.2% of the variance in caring (Duffy et al., 2007). Patients in this sample perceived nurses as caring when they were responsive to their families and allowed them to be engaged in the health care situation, including decision making. Other nursing theorists have spoken to the importance of families (Johnson, 1980; King, 2001; Watson, 1979), and the empirical literature is pointing to family involvement as an important component to patient healing (Campbell & Rudisill, 2006; Mangurten et al., 2006). Why is it, then, that patients are often marginalized from their significant others during hospitalization? Whose interests are nurses serving?

The importance of families to the health and well-being of patients, particularly those who are hospitalized, is well recognized by pediatric, obstetric, rehabilitation, psychiatric, and oncology nurses and associated health care facilities. For example, round-the-clock visitation, routine family meetings, and resources geared to the needs of family members are commonplace. Using these examples, nurses in all health care settings can appreciate and involve families as they care for ill persons.

These eight caring factors originated from Watson's (1979, 1985) original work and were validated more recently in a study of 557 adults in 5 acute care institutions. Although limited by the sample and the setting, the findings provided some support for Watson's and other nursing theorists' views of nursing and were congruent with preliminary evidence. The factors are not necessarily used all at once or in equal fashion; rather, the individual patient and the situation inform the nurse in their appropriate use.

To that end, caring relationships can be viewed as multifaceted, comprised of several factors, and, when applied, induce positive feelings in recipients. In fact, the recipient's reaction to a caring nurse is crucial because it is this emotion that guides future interactions (and thus, the outcomes of care). In other words, the patient's ability to progress is mediated somewhat by the feelings generated as a consequence of caring relationships.

When the nurse authentically cares (versus acting out of obligation or mechanistically), positive attitudes are generated in the recipient (see Figure 4.2).

The nurse in Figure 4.2 is pictured as an octagon (simulating the eight caring factors). As he/she relates to the patient in a caring manner, the patient registers that the help provided was genuine and sincere (and he/she feels "cared for"). This positive emotion allows the patient to relax and feel noticed and secure; it provides the foundation and leads the way to future caring interactions. Relationships comprised of the caring factors benefit not only patients but nurses themselves because sharing oneself with another in an authentic mode is consciousness-raising; one learns and grows as a human in caring relationships.

In an earlier work, Duffy (2003) spoke to the phases of caring relationships (see Figure 4.3). Through the process of interaction, patients and nurses come together, communicate, and mutually express themselves. Over time, an authentic connection occurs that deepens the patient–nurse relationship beyond the two persons. In fact, in a genuine connection, the nurse recognizes his/herself in the other. Watson (1979, 1985) calls this type of relationship *transpersonal.* Through sustained connection, the other becomes *known;* the relationship transcends time and intensifies to the point that allows the nurse to design unique interventions and even foresee patient and family needs. Knowing another provides the insight to detect potential problems early, to be protective,

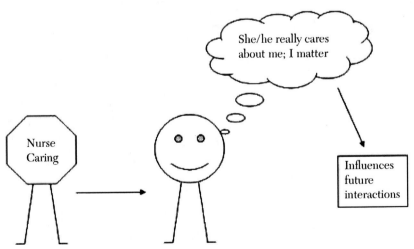

Figure 4.2 Recipients' reaction to nurse caring.

to allow anticipatory guidance and creative problem solving, and to facilitate healthy behaviors. This knowing phase is dependent on prior interaction and connection and influences future interaction. The phases are dynamic and often overlap; they inform succeeding phases.

Effective use of the caring factors requires integration of external forces (education, experience, current research, role-modeling) with internal awareness (self-knowledge). However, working in this manner is somewhat countercultural in this day of fast-paced, highly intense health care environments. As such, it requires the ability to tolerate some uncertainty or ambiguity, remaining attentive and open-minded, and the courage to advocate for the expression of the caring factors as crucial to quality nursing care. Use of oneself in this way honors the individual and the profession of nursing as a life-giving energy source. Using the caring factors through the interaction, connection, and knowing phases of caring relationships is the cornerstone of nursing that guides the implementation of all other activities.

THE PRACTICE OF NURSING USING THE QUALITY-CARING MODEL©

The practice of professional nursing is essential to quality health outcomes. It is the one continuous and stabilizing force in acute care institu-

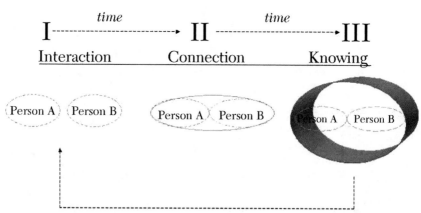

Figure 4.3 Phases of caring relationships.
From "Caring Relationships and Evidence-Based Practice: Can They Co-Exist?" by J. Duffy, 2003, *International Journal of Human Caring, 7*(3), 45–49.

tions that is available to patients and families 24 hours a day. Performing nursing according to a nursing model provides a foundation for decision making, nursing control over practice, direction for daily activities, and research and evaluation (see Table 4.2).

The Quality-Caring Model provides the practitioner with a set of concepts, parameters, and specific behaviors that guide thoughts and actions. First, it provides direction regarding human beings in terms of their relationships and considers these relationships necessary for human advancement. When a person seeks health care, his/her relationship-nature is extended to the health care situation and the nurse. The nurse, using his/her own self-knowledge together with other worldly information, interacts in a caring manner to engage the person in health-related matters. Effective use of the caring factors enables the patient–nurse relationship to transcend person and time adding a depth or third dimension that enhances the lives of both individuals.

Following the well-known nursing process (Yura & Walsh, 1967), assessment is holistic with equal attention to all components of the human condition. The plan of care reflects *both* physical and psychosocialcul-turalspiritual issues and addresses them using the caring factors. These factors are independent functions of the nurse and presume ongoing interaction. The interaction is reciprocal and honors both individuals

Table 4.2

BENEFITS OF A PROFESSIONAL PRACTICE MODEL

1. Nursing values provide the foundation for practice
2. RN control over practice decisions (autonomy)
3. Enhanced clinical outcomes
4. Shared leadership—RNs actively participate and have meaningful impact on decisions
5. RN responsibility and accountability for high-quality nursing practice within the realm of the nurse practice act
6. The model drives patient care
7. The model is used as a basis for research and evaluation of nursing care
8. Improved image of nursing
9. Enhanced RN job satisfaction

as unique and worthy of attention. Implementing the plan of care is accomplished in mutual interaction with patients and families and collaboratively with other health professionals; the caring factors remain the cornerstone of all transactions. Nurses' primary role in this process is the creation and maintenance of caring relationships. Finally, evaluating care using the Quality-Caring Model is both formative (ongoing) and summative (cumulative). During the provision of care, nurses through caring relationships validate patients' progression toward health and revise care in collaboration with the patient and other health care providers. Throughout the process, nursing-sensitive outcomes such as comfort, functional status, knowledge, maintenance of human dignity, and safety are assessed to learn how well the patient's needs were met and to inform future nursing practice.

A special consideration in the Quality-Caring Model is the dimension of time. It is considered a necessary aspect of caring relationships. Nurses are conditioned to being alert to signs and symptoms of future problems; such anticipation along with the many tasks required during an 8- or 12-hour shift keeps nurses' attention always on the future. In this busyness the nurse often is trying to get somewhere or finish something in order to move on to the next task. Such a hurried, frantic pace makes present situations seem like impediments that can create impatience and frustration. All too often nurses are so lost in the *doing* that the *being* (caring) of the profession is forgotten. Frequently, nurses are overheard saying, "There is never enough time."

Another way to view this dilemma is to consider how nurses allocate the time they have. The reality of clock time and tasks (doing) are important to quality patient care, but so is the present moment (being). It is in such moments that patients need to be heard, their pain comforted, their dignity honored. Furthermore, nurses as humans need to access that inner quiet found deep within often during the work shift to remember who they are (caring) and the meaning of their work. When nurses' caring essence is balanced with their doing, a higher-quality nursing care is rendered. Imagine a busy nurse who has an intravenous catheter dripping the caring factors into him/her during a work shift. While the actions/tasks may not change, *how* they are implemented will be different.

Consider the following example.

> I was assigned to take care of Mrs. Edy, a 55-year-old Caucasian woman who was scheduled for a revision of her colostomy. She had colon cancer

and this was the third revision. Apparently, it was leaking and infected. I had 4 other patients but during the admission process, we connected right away. As I was taking the history, I let her go on for a little while about her work as an accountant and her family. This allowed me to know her as a person not just "a case" going for surgery on our unit. I noticed her facial expressions as she talked; she was grimacing and frowning. I listened carefully to her story while she shared that she is tired of the same surgery and wonders if it will "work" this time. Settling her in her bed, I clarified the procedure and the skill of the surgeon and then arranged her environment so that she felt at ease (pointing out my phone number, how the bathroom works, etc). She continued to talk and eventually shared that she wanted to be home for Christmas because her grandson was coming to visit. During the physical assessment, I noticed her abdominal scars and then I saw the colostomy for the first time. I was disgusted at its appearance and smell. Mrs. Edy sensed my emotions and looked away saying how this surgery has humiliated her. She continued to say, "If only you knew me when I was well. I am no longer the same woman!" I asked how she is different. She says that she no longer can relate physically to her husband and feels useless as a woman. Using gentle touch and eye contact, I redressed the colostomy. Then I asked her if she would like to talk to another woman who had a colostomy for colon cancer. She replied, "Maybe after my surgery." After the assessment, as I was charting in the room, I asked her to tell me about her grandson. That was when she asked me if I had any children. I told her that I was looking forward to going home for my daughter's 3rd birthday party. As I left her room, I thought about the courageousness of this woman who, although a little downhearted, continued to relate well to other human beings. I drew some strength for myself through this interaction.

The next afternoon, I was completing her post-op vital signs and dressing checks and found her crying. During our interaction, she relayed to me her sadness about not being able to see her grandson grow up. I probed a little to find out what she knew about her illness and found out that she assumed from hearing of others that she would die within 6 months! I briefly checked on my other 4 patients and then returned to her room. Using this opportunity, I suggested that we peruse together the literature (on the cancer unit) to see what options she had vis à vis treatment. When I went out to the nurses' station, I checked her chart to see what the surgeon and oncologist had written about her cancer prognosis. Finding a decent prognosis (at least for the short term), I later discussed the information I had learned with Mrs. Edy. I found that she really did not understand her prognosis; during rounds, I asked her oncologist to talk to her and really explain what she had to look forward to. As I was reflecting about Mrs. Edy on my way home from work, I felt happy with myself that perhaps I helped her rearrange her thinking about her illness. I also wondered how I would think if I had this disease.

This example occurred on a busy surgical floor; can you identify the caring factors the nurse used? Although this nurse had many tasks to accomplish, she understood that this moment with this patient was primary. As she worked efficiently to complete the admission assessment and dress an offensive wound, she initiated a caring relationship by using several caring factors (human respect, attentive reassurance, healing environment) that allowed Mrs. Edy the freedom to express herself. The nurse, during a routine post-op assessment, used the caring relationship she initiated the prior day to help Mrs. Edy understand that her illness was not necessarily an immediate death sentence (mutual problem solving) and went on to involve her physician. While the tasks she performed were similar in nature to other nurses, this nurse added the depth of caring to enrich the experience and both parties benefited.

Now consider the following example.

Mr. Malone was a 69-year-old male admitted to an oncology unit with late stage large cell lung cancer. He was somewhat short of breath with O2 sats at 81. CXR revealed the tumor had invaded large portions of his lung parenchyma. He was placed on the oncology unit with a 100% rebreather mask. He had five children, one of whom was a nurse. His condition did not improve and his nurse-daughter advocated for a DNR order. His secretions increasingly became worse and dilaudid was considered. Although his daughter remained with him throughout the night, she rang the bell often for doses of IV Dilaudid to help his cough and breathing. I had 6 patients and had all I could do to keep up with the constant medicating of Mr. Malone. So I medicated him each time and then left the room to let Mr. Malone and his daughter have privacy. This went on all night until he needed the medication every 20 minutes or so. At 4:30 A.M. the daughter suggested that maybe an IV drip would be advantageous. Since it was close to change of shift I thought it best to discuss this with the day nurse who would see the physician on rounds. At 7:30 A.M. the physician made rounds and found Mr. Malone's lung fields to be filled with fluid—he ordered Lasix and the daughter asked him about starting low dose Dilaudid I.V. to ease his discomfort. The physician agreed . . .

The day nurse came in around 9 A.M. and asked the daughter "if she know what was going on?" The daughter understood the gravity of her father's condition and wanted to ensure his comfort during the dying process by maintaining a consistent Dilaudid level. However, she did not want to "snow" her father or cause lasting Dilaudid-induced side effects for there was still some unfinished family business. The nurse brought the Dilaudid drip in and immediately set it at 4MG where it remained throughout the day. The nurse came in around 1 P.M., observed the situation and left. Mr. Malone was visited that evening by the priest (whom his daughter called), his wife, and his other children. As I came on the night shift I saw Mr. Malone surrounded by his wife and children through the door. Since the daughter who was a nurse was present and I had five other patients who were more aggressively ill, I attended to them. After all, Mr. Malone was a DNR, and he was comfortable. At 7:22 A.M., the daughter came out to the nurses' station to announce that her father had expired. I called the resident to do the pronouncement. We cleaned him up, although the daughter had already removed his rebreather mask, and sent him to the morgue. I felt heavy hearted as I left work that morning.

This example occurred on a busy oncology unit. What caring factors are present? How would you rate Mr. Malone's nursing care? The narrative provides a view of a busy nurse doing the best she can to care for several patients. Despite this fact, Mr. Malone and his family are important persons with a crucial life situation facing them. They are focused on his dying process and the impending loss to the family and do not understand the workload of the nurse. Should they? Can you suggest alternative ways the nurse could have related to this patient and his family?

The two preceding illustrations of nursing practice were provided to demonstrate how the use of caring factors attends to the intrinsic value of both patients and nurses. In the first instance, the nurse used several caring factors during the admission process to gather facts, engage the patient, and set the stage for future interactions. Moreover, she left the patient with her dignity intact and with some encouragement for the immediate future. On the next day, the patient felt comfortable opening up to the nurse and through mutual problem solving, the nurse was able to help the patient think differently about her illness. In the second example, the nurse did not engage the patient or the daughter. In fact, she doesn't even relay whether the patient was conscious! She is very concerned about all her patients, but in her busyness, she doesn't see the person who is dying at this moment and how that is impacting his daughter. She remains detached from him (unconscious) and is driven by the many tasks she has to accomplish during her shift.

How do these nursing situations impact the nurse? The first feels strengthened after the interaction with Mrs. Edy, but the second nurse is gloomy and sullen. *Doing*, even if one completes all tasks, is never enough if *being* is not at the core of the actions. The Quality-Caring

Model centers on the *being* of nursing practice for it is proposed as the key to caring relationships. Use of the caring factors throughout the nursing process changes the paradigm of nursing from biomedical procedures to holistic caring relationships that advance human systems. Imagine the collective practice of nursing where all nurses are authentically present to themselves and their patients!

SUMMARY

The impact of illness on patients and families was highlighted in this chapter with special emphasis on the threats to personal meanings and how the health care system can sometimes add to suffering. Caring intention as a prerequisite to actual behavior was differentiated from the desire to care and develops through one's lived experiences. Specific attitudes and meanings of caring attained through experience, formal learning, self-reflecting, and observing others comprise one's intention to care. Such intention generates positive behaviors on the part of the nurse. Eight caring factors, preliminarily validated through research, were explained in detail with examples provided. It is hypothesized that use of these factors engenders positive feelings in the recipient that informs future interactions and advancement toward health. Acting in this manner also benefits the nurse in terms of professional growth. Using the Quality-Caring Model in practice was explained with special emphasis on the time dimension. The importance of balancing *doing* with *being* creates a higher-quality nursing care that can be delivered. Two contrasting examples provide a more in-depth glimpse of the Quality-Caring Model in action. Nursing is presented as a blend of doing and being that raises the holistic nature of humans (nurses and patients) to a higher level.

CALLS TO ACTION

Illness exposes patients and their families to threats—physiological, societal, and personal—that render them vulnerable. The health care system unknowingly adds to this risk by setting up the conditions for adverse outcomes. **Eliminate** one condition at your

(continued)

institution that could influence adverse outcomes for patients, families, or students.

Aware, fully integrated persons are more apt to direct their intentions toward another in a caring manner; resulting behaviors become more genuine. **Read** Schlitz, M. M., Vieten, C., & Amorok, T. (2007). *Living deeply: The art and science of transformation in everyday life.* Oakland, CA: New Harbinger Publications, Inc.

Keeping in mind that human persons who are ill (regardless of their age, physical or mental capacity, or social status) are mothers, fathers, sons, daughters, grandmothers and grandfathers, hold societal roles, and are members of unique communities is crucial. Viewing patients this way, in spite of their weakened state, helps nurses to appreciate the totality of patients, including their significance to others. Observing and remaining conscious—even taking pleasure in patients' roles and responsibilities when they are not ill— preserves their honor. **Get more information** about your patients' roles and responsibilities in their families and their communities.

The caring factors, when used expertly, facilitate a different form of patient–nurse relationship. This transformed relationship goes beyond person and time, adding a third dimension, depth, that enriches the lives of both individuals. **Master** the caring factors.

The duality of doing (tasks) and being (authentic use of self in the moment) at the same time is crucial to quality patient care. Nurses who integrate the two create meaning, are comforting, and affirm human dignity. **Practice** being and doing together.

Reflective Questions/Applications for Students

1. Discuss how a pediatric patient who is hospitalized for acute asthma can alter the family system.
2. Consider the last patient you took care of. How do you think the experience of illness (or health) altered this person's view of his/her self?

3. Explain the word *intention*. What lived experiences can you point to that informed your caring intention?

4. Using a real patient situation, describe how the caring factors could have been used to enrich the patient and family experience.

5. Describe the phases of caring relationships. Provide examples of each phase.

6. Answer the following questions.

   - In what ways does the timing of baths/daily weights/assessments at your institution honor the individual needs of patients?

   - What proactive measures do you engage in to assist patients with pain relief?

   - How do you center yourself in order to focus with intention on patient/families?

   - In what ways do you demonstrate knowledge and awareness of caring principles?

   - Do you make professional decisions in the best interest of patients/families?

7. Using the case of Mr. Malone, answer the following questions. Who was the patient? Did Mr. Malone receive *professional* nursing care? Why or why not?

Reflective Questions/Applications for Educators

8. How would you sensitize nursing students to the vulnerabilities of illness?

9. What teaching strategies are effective for integrating caring factors with technical skills?

10. When should the caring factors be taught in a four-year undergraduate program? A graduate program? What about an Associates Degree program?

Reflective Questions/Applications for Nurse Leaders

11. Beginning with the admission assessment, does nursing practice in your organization require revision?

12. What is the best way to engage staff nurses in discussions about the caring factors?

13.   What family visitation policies exist at your institution? Do they take into consideration the affiliation needs as stated in the Quality-Caring Model?

14.   How do you know your patients feel "cared for?"

REFERENCES

American Nurses Association. (2001). *Code of ethics for nurses with interpretive statements.* Silver Springs, MD: American Nurses Publishing.

Boykin, A., & Schoenhofer, S. (1993). *Nursing as caring: A model for transforming practice.* New York: National League for Nursing Press.

Campbell, P., & Rudisill, P. (2006). Psychosocial needs of the critically ill obstetric patient: The nurse's role. *Critical Care Nursing Quarterly, 29*(10), 77–80.

Center for Disease Control and Prevention. (2003). *National Center for Health Statistics, National Hospital Discharge survey. Table 95.* Retrieved October 4, 2004, from http://.cdc.gov/nchs/data/hus/tables/2003/03hus095.pdf

Center for Disease Control and Prevention. (2004). *Injuries among older adults.* Retrieved October 5, 2004, from http://www.cdc.gov/ncipc/olderadults.htm

Chang, E., Hancock, K., Chenoweth, L., Jeon, Y., Glasson, J., Gradidge, K., et al. (2003). The influence of demographic variables and ward type on elderly patients' perceptions of needs and satisfaction during hospitalization. *International Journal of Nursing Practice, 9*(3), 191–201.

Chopra, D. (2004). *The book of secrets.* New York: Three Rivers Press.

Duffy, J. (2003). Caring relationships and evidence-based practice: Can they coexist? *International Journal of Human Caring, 7*(3), 45–50.

Duffy, J. R., & Hoskins, L. M. (2003). The quality-caring model-blending dual paradigms. *Advances in Nursing Science, 26*(1), 77–88.

Duffy, J., Hoskins, L. M., & Seifert, R. F. (2007). Dimensions of caring: Psychometric evaluation of the caring assessment tool. *Advances of Nursing Science, 30*(3), 235–245.

Fishbein, M., & Ajzen, I. (1975). *Belief, attitude, intention, and behavior: An introduction to theory and research.* Reading, MA: Addison-Wesley.

Husserl, E. (1980). *Phenomenology and the foundations of the sciences.* Translated by T. E. Klein, Jr., & W. E. Pohl. The Hague, Netherlands: Martinus Nijhoff.

Institute for Healthcare Improvement. (2008). Retrieved February 27, 2008, from http://www.ihi.org/IHI/Topics/PatientSafety/SafetyGeneral/changes/Develop+a+Culture+of+Safety.htm

Institute of Medicine. (2001). *Crossing the quality chasm.* Washington, DC: National Academy Press.

Institute of Medicine. (2004). *Keeping patients safe: Transforming the work environment of nurses.* Washington, DC: Author.

Johnson, D. E. (1980). The behavioral system model for nursing. In J. P. Riehl & C. Roy (Eds.), *Conceptual models for nursing practice* (2nd ed., pp. 207–216). New York: Appleton-Century-Crofts.

King, I. M. (2001). Theory of goal attainment. In M. Parker (Ed.), *Nursing theories and nursing practice* (pp. 275–286). Philadelphia, PA: Davis.

Mangurten, J., Scott, S., Guzzetta, C., Clark, A. P., Vinson, L., Sperry, J., et al. (2006). Effects of family presence during resuscitation and invasive procedures in a pediatric emergency department. *Journal of Emergency Nursing, 32*(3), 225–233.

Maslow, A. (1954). *Motivation and personality.* New York: Harper.

Maslow, A. (1971). *The farther reaches of human nature.* New York: The Viking Press.

Nightingale, F. (1992). *Notes on nursing: What it is and what it is not* (Com. Ed.). Philadelphia, PA: Lippincott. (Originally published in 1859.)

Peplau, H. E. (1988). *Interpersonal relations in nursing.* New York: Springer Publishing.

Perugini, M., & Bagozzi, R. P. (2004). The distinction between desires and intentions. *European Journal of Social Psychology, 34,* 69–84.

Rogers, C. (1961). On becoming a person. *Archives of General Psychiatry, 62,* 1377–1384.

Sager, M., & Rudberg, M. (1998). Functional decline associated with hospitalization for acute illness. *Clinics in Geriatric Medicine, 14*(4), 669–679.

Swanson, K. M. (1991). Empirical development of a middle-range theory of caring. *Nursing Research, 40*(3), 161–166.

Topf, M., & Thompson, S. (2001). Interactive relationships between hospital patients' noise-induced stress and other stress with sleep. *Heart and Lung, 30*(4), 237–243.

Watson, J. (1979). *Nursing: The philosophy and science of caring.* Boston: Little, Brown and Company.

Watson, J. (1985). *Nursing: Human science and human care.* Norwalk, CT: Appleton-Century-Crofts.

Watson, J. (1999). *Postmodern nursing and beyond.* Edinburgh, Scotland: Churchill Livingstone.

Watson, J. (2006). *Theory evolution.* Retrieved December 3, 2007, from http://hschealth.uchsc.edu/son/faculty/jw_evolution.htm

Williams, A. (2004). Patients with comorbidities: Perceptions of acute care services. *Journal of Advanced Nursing, 46*(1), 13–22.

Williams, A., & Irurita, V. (2004). Therapeutic and non-therapeutic interpersonal interactions: The patient's perspective. *Journal of Clinical Nursing, 13,* 806–815.

Wolf, Z. R., Zuelo, P. R., Goldberg, E., Crowthers, R., & Jacobson, N. (2006). The caring behaviors inventory for elders: Development and psychometric characteristics. *International Journal of Human Caring, 10*(1), 49–59.

Yalom, I. D. (1975). *The theory and practice of group psychotherapy.* New York: Basic Books.

Yura, H., & Walsh, M. B. (1967). *The nursing process: Assessing, planning, implementing, evaluating.* New York: Appleton-Century-Crofts.

5   Caring for Each Other

Coming together is a beginning. Keeping together is progress. Working together is success.

—Henry Ford

Keywords: **collegial relationships, collaborative relationships, interprofessional practice**

THE CRITICAL CHALLENGE OF COLLEAGUESHIP

Professional nurses today are a multigenerational, diverse working group with individual psychosocioculturalspiritual characteristics. In addition, they are caring for the most complex, diverse, acute, and chronically ill population this nation has ever seen. They supervise un-licensed personnel, chase down equipment and supplies, coordinate health care teams, sort through and document on numerous medical records, and are overwhelmed by tasks. Meanwhile, the economic con-straints of managed care have forced hospitals to concentrate on cost containment and restructuring efforts, many of which have resulted in overworked professional nurses. Acute care professional nurses today are frequently working at the interface between the efficiency needs of the health care system and the human caring needs of the populations they serve. In this environment, there is enormous responsibility, high intensity, and workplace tension.

Complicating these system difficulties are nursing-specific concerns that plague the workforce. Currently, hospitals have an estimated 116,000 registered nurse vacancies and by 2020, the United States will face a projected shortage of one million registered nurses (American Hospital Association, 2008). Younger nurses are demanding more flexible work schedules, while others still are choosing careers outside of nursing altogether. Furthermore, recruitment and retention issues, intershift conflict, and nurse scheduling practices prohibit continuity of care. Finally, there are tremendous pressures to conform to the system and "pay your dues."

To make matters worse, intraprofessional insensitivities exist in practice, administration, and academia. Horizontal violence among peers is sadly prevalent and includes gossiping, insults, sabotaging behavior, isolating behaviors, and even creating uneven work assignments (Christmas, 2007). Disrespect and lack of support, verbal abuse (Ferns & Meerabeau, 2008), violence, and even bullying tactics have appeared in the recent literature (Lewis, 2006). These activities can take many forms, from deliberate lying to blaming, manipulation, and aggressive acts in the workplace. In one qualitative study of nursing intraprofessional relationships, the findings indicated that over time many nurses become resilient to the effect of interpersonal workplace conflict (Duddle & Boughton, 2007). Furthermore, nursing managers are often at a loss at how to intervene during such conflicts, and many times they are the source of them. In nursing education, studies of incivility in both students and faculty are discouraging (Clark, 2007, 2008; Ehrmann, 2005).

One example of such behavior recently occurred in an acute care hospital. Two nurses at shift report were angrily yelling at each other in the nurses' station regarding the assignment of the oncoming nurse. This occurred during the early morning hours and was witnessed by new graduates, students, patients and families, physicians, and other RNs. The verbal abuse was profound and escalated to a level that was extremely unprofessional. Sadly, no one intervened, and it lasted several minutes, disrupting the unit and leaving bad feelings, especially among the new graduate nurses.

Another example from academia occurred in a midsized school of nursing. A young faculty member who was writing a proposal for funding asked a senior, tenured professor to review her application and offer suggestions for improvement. While the more senior professor indicated she would gladly critique the young professor's work, she returned it within 20 minutes with a couple of spelling errors highlighted. It was obvious that the senior professor did not take this request seriously, and the younger professor was left without the guidance she needed to submit her proposal; one might even go so far as to say that she was sabotaged. The senior professor verbally indicated her willingness to help but nonverbally did not complete the work. Such actions do not generate feelings of "being cared for"; rather, they harm future interactions. Working this way goes against the norms of the profession and can be a source of ongoing conflict for nurses. Furthermore, Marshall and Robson (2005) report that such conflict often goes unacknowledged, resulting in mistrust and anxiety that are significant contributors to unsafe work cultures.

Ordinarily, in the work environment, members of a similar profession are known as colleagues. The word *colleagueship*, however, has a deeper meaning and speaks to respect for a fellow colleague's contribution to the work. The Minnesota Nurses Association (1999), in their position statement *Colleagueship in Nursing Practice*, highlights that nurses individually and collectively display collegial behaviors when they reach mutual agreements regarding patient care, consult with each other, and collaboratively create environments that sustain professional growth.

COLLABORATIVE RELATIONSHIPS

Professional nurses are already connected to one another by the common bond of caring for patients and families and the many nursing-specific practices and artifacts that dominate the profession. This connection offers a unique opportunity for nurses to come together and, through caring, create higher-level expressions of human interaction. While colleagues typically are associated through common work, *being collaborative* has a stronger meaning. It denotes a commitment to working together—sharing knowledge, observing role models, making decisions together, rooting for one another—these are all ways that professional nurses demonstrate a collaborative nature. *Being collaborative* suggests a higher form of relating to another such that mutual goals are attained (in this case, what's in the best interest of the patient and family).

Collaboration is an advanced form of relating that requires intention, ongoing interaction, connection, and knowing the other, similar to the phases of caring nurses' use with patients. True collaboration is a process initiated in relationships that, when nurtured (using the caring factors) over time, enable shared responsibility and decision making for patient care. The nature of relationships among professional nurses can advance or hinder patient and family outcomes as well as the profession.

Just as nurses' progress through the phases of caring relationships with patients and families, so too do they advance caring relationships with fellow nurses and other health professionals. Using the caring factors and interacting frequently over time, deeper connections form that advance to knowing the other. When one is *known*, interactions become more natural and supportive. Oftentimes, responsibilities are shared and projects implemented that support the progress of the partners.

One pivotal relationship that appears frequently in the literature is the nurse–physician relationship. In the acute care area in particular, this relationship is crucial to the delivery of safe and quality patient care. Several studies have linked improved patient outcomes and improved nurse satisfaction to collaborative nurse–physician relationships (Baggs, Ryan, Phelps, Richeson, & Johnson, 1992; Knaus, Draper, Wagner, & Zimmerman, 1986; Scott, Sochalski, & Aiken, 1999; Shortell, Rosseau, Gillies, Devers, & Simons, 1992). As nurses and physicians interact through open communication, they share common tasks, seek the opinions of the other, and work cohesively for the benefit of the patient and family. Collaboration is a genuine process that preserves the professional identity and humanness of the partners. Just as self-knowing/caring and use of the caring factors enhances the patient–nurse and nurse–nurse relationships, so too do they influence the nurse–physician relationship. Genuine collaborative relationships break down walls of separation between health care providers and form interdependencies among them that positively influence patients. The Quality-Caring Model© asserts that nurses accept responsibility for and implement healthy, caring interpersonal relationships with each other and members of the health care team. Doing so has the potential to enhance patient outcomes, affirm each health care team member's unique contribution, and increase work satisfaction.

A CARING APPROACH TO INTERPROFESSIONAL PRACTICE

"Interprofessional practice refers to a highly integrated framework for collaboration among professionals" (Geva, Barsky, & Westernoff, 2000, p. 3). Through patient and family assessments and interventions, professionals develop common objectives for the work, and then, through the process of authentic collaboration (a form of caring), a consensus develops in terms of a shared treatment plan. This approach uses a "we" versus an "I" frame of reference and works best when the professionals can think broadly (systems thinking) and in a learning mode. And, if taken to the ultimate level, the patient and family are considered part of the team. One good tool for performing this way is evidence-based practice—it shares a common language and is oriented toward what's best for the patient. Although emerging from interprofessional education, interprofessional practice (IP) is a natural next step in the improvement of services for complex patients and families.

Just as patients and families have unique characteristics, so too do members of the health care team. In the workplace, health care team members bring their unique life experiences, including the psychosocioculturalspiritual perspectives that define them. They also have specific educational and credentialing backgrounds that ground their practice. For example, one source in England reported that physician-initiated interactions focused on *giving information* or instructions, while nurse-initiated interactions took on the form of *requesting information* or orders (Reeves & Lewin, 2004). These are behaviors based on old roles where nursing was considered a part of medicine versus its own complementary profession. These differing perspectives can be a source of frustration when power or politics (turf wars) get in the way, or they can provide a more holistic perspective from which to deliver high-quality patient care. Thus, crucial to providing high-quality care is the affirmation and appreciation of each other's unique scope of practice and contribution. Using the caring factors nurses are so intimate with can assist in initiating, cultivating, and sustaining the collaborative relationships necessary for IP.

Mutual problem solving includes conferring about how best to approach the patient and solve his/her health problems. Helping each other understand, exploring alternative approaches, brainstorming together, and checking in with each other provide the foundation for expert care. Accepting constructive feedback and experimenting with different ways to provide care are also important collaborative behaviors. Implicit in this factor is the ability of nurses to seek out other health care providers, including physicians, to learn their views and goals for patient care. Making the effort to participate with physicians on patient rounds is an example of this behavior.

Using *attentive reassurance* with other health professionals implies accessibility and optimism. Slowing down enough to notice the other and confidently work together is enriching. Displaying behaviors that suggest acceptance such as calling the other by name is a demonstration of *human respect,* another caring factor that enhances the relationship. Conveying an *encouraging manner* that is enthusiastic and supportive can instill trust and belief in the other. *Appreciating the unique meanings* that each health care provider brings to the health care situation lets the other know the importance of his/her role and helps them feel understood.

Creating a *healing environment* as it relates to interprofessional practice considers the setting where patient care is taking place and the factors related to employee privacy and safety. It also refers to features such as the appropriate norms of behavior. The dominant biomedical, highly intense, and rushed physical environment of acute care does not always promote full attention on human beings, including other, open communication, and sharing of ideas.

> Nurses set the tone on patient care units and can "make or break" other health care providers as they try to deliver care. Just imagine July 1st in academic health centers where all the new interns are facing their first real assignments. Nurses can facilitate their transition or thwart it. Creating an atmosphere where these young physicians feel at home on a particular department and are communicated with as valued team members can ease the way for them as well as provide the groundwork for future nurse–physician relationships. Taking the responsibility to ensure a safe and private place to practice and creating a culture of teamwork are caring behaviors that fall within the realm of professional nursing.

A good example of taking responsibility for the practice on a unit was recently reported by Carter et al. (2008). Nurses on a particular unit were concerned that the new graduates were so focused on their list of activities to be accomplished that caring behaviors were devalued, thus creating a task-oriented versus the more preferable person-oriented environment. They acted on their observations and completed a study using focus group methodology to compare patients' and nurses' caring perceptions. Findings included that "caring for each other was essential to keep staff energized and able to work lovingly with patients" (p. 57). They then used these data to invigorate the nursing staff using several initiatives.

Basic human needs and *affiliation needs* are important to health care providers as well as patients. Ensuring fellow nurses get to lunch or take bathroom breaks, working with each other for special scheduling needs, and remembering to affirm each other honor the humanness of us all.

Using the caring factors as a framework for IP sets the tone for future interactions and creates positive emotions that generate ease in the work setting. The many professions involved in patient care share responsibility, lessening individual stress and burden. Professional nurses who are experts in caring can make the difference in interprofessional practice.

USING THE QUALITY-CARING MODEL TO ADVANCE INTERPROFESSIONAL PRACTICE

Caring for each other nurse to nurse and interprofessionally is essential to quality health outcomes. It is depicted in the Quality-Caring Model as an integral relationship and has benefits not only for the patient and family but for health care providers as well. As a group of like-minded professionals seeking to care for patients in need, the integrated nurse (one who has balanced his/her self-knowledge together with worldly knowledge) who uses the caring factors enables collaborative relationships to flourish.

Seeking out other health professionals, willingly sharing assessment data, asking for clarification, actively listening to explanations, participating in patient care rounds or performance improvement meetings, keeping each other apprised of changes in conditions, *being* collaborative, making suggestions, and accepting feedback are all collaborative caring behaviors.

Consider the following example:

A young 29-year-old couple who had just given birth to their firstborn were recovering on a postpartum unit of a large Magnet (American Hospital Association, 2008) hospital in the Midwest. As described by them, "The pediatrician made a point of telling us many times to keep the infant on his back. A very overbearing nurse kept placing the child on his side. When the father asked about the discrepancy, the nurse said that 'side-lying is a tradition that I find best.' Confused, the father asked the pediatrician who said, 'I know . . . we fight with the nurses all the time about this.' In addition, when the pediatrician asked this nurse for the results of the bilirubin test she ordered, the nurse said, 'You didn't order it.' The pediatrician went over to the computer, found the order, and relayed her findings to the nurse. The nurse then hurried on out to complete the order. The pediatrician commented, 'Sometimes, I just don't get it.'" The couple relayed that this tension between the professions caused them to lose confidence in the nurse, and it affected all the remaining interactions with her. Although these examples don't seem like big issues, the couple found it unnecessary and frightening to the point that they "didn't allow the baby out of my sight." It was obvious to them that the physicians and nurses did not get along, were untrustworthy, and inconsistent in their instructions. This added to their stress and caused bad feelings.

While this example is unfortunate, others exist that show positive collaboration among professionals and highlight how this impacts outcomes. At the Washington Hospital Center in Washington, DC, for example, a performance improvement initiative comprised of nursing staff, physicians, respiratory therapy, a social worker, pharmacists, nutrition support care, spiritual care, utilization review staff, the patient advocate, and infection control was formed on a medical intensive care unit to facilitate joint protocols and practices. Creative interventions were developed by the team addressing patients who were extubated, sedated, or were experiencing long-term ventilator weaning. Daily goal sheets and a specialty cart were used to keep everyone focused. Champions were appointed for each protocol, the team was educated together, and the entire team held the group accountable. Despite the fact that an increased number of mechanically ventilated patients were admitted to the unit, a decrease in overall length of stay from 6.2 to 3.6 days was realized. The mechanically ventilated patients' mean length of stay decreased from 9.5 to 6 days, and mortality decreased from 36% to 23%. Even more impressive, ventilator-associated pneumonia consistently remained below the Center for Disease Control's (CDC's) 50th percentile. Implementing these initiatives in the medical intensive care unit saved the organization $8 million per year. This group also tackled a catheter-related bloodstream infection rate (CR-BSI) consistently above the CDC's 90th percentile. As a result of information gained at an international symposium, staff introduced the idea of a central line insertion bundle to the unit's Performance Improvement Committee. The bundle consisted of a partnership between nurses and physicians using a checklist that prompts adherence, physician education on central line technique and site selection, assisted central line insertion (two-person procedure—RN observer) with equipment cart and checklist, maximum barrier protection, procedural pause, and empowerment and accountability of the RN to stop the procedure for any breaks in technique. Unit-based CR-BSI rates were posted monthly and discussed in staff meetings. Collaboration between the Infection Control Department and nursing identified a nurse champion for the bundle and an infection control liaison to report isolation status and necessary precautions for all patients daily. Each day on rounds, all central venous catheters were evaluated for necessity, site, and catheter day. This collaboration between multiple health care professionals resulted in a decrease in primary bloodstream infections per 1,000 catheter days from 18 to 0!

Another example of positive collaboration among colleagues occurred in a public health study in which nurses and teachers collaborated on an instructional program on farm safety for use in high schools (Reed & Kidd, 2004). While problems in recruitment hampered the two-group controlled design, findings demonstrated the benefit of the program. Of importance to this discussion is the genuine collaboration between secondary school teachers and nurse researchers; working together they were able to enrich the curriculum.

Another innovative program, the *Workforce Environment (WE) Governance Board,* was developed in an academic-service partnership model to meet the goals of improving the RN work environment and improving selected patient outcomes (Latham, Hogan, & Ringl, 2008). Through a mentoring program, the authors built a team of informal leaders who would serve to change the unit culture to one of positive and relational support. An improved relationship between academia and health care service included mutual respect and improved resource sharing. The university adopted course content, and the nurse-to-nurse support fostered in this program improved the workplace environment.

Using forums such as "Schwartz Rounds" to openly dialogue about the struggles that health professionals share in specific patient situations has offered participating institutions an avenue for better understanding and compassion (The Kenneth B. Schwartz Center, 2007). Finally, working together to improve and accelerate clinical science offers health care professionals opportunities to test common conceptual frameworks (Grey & Connolly, 2008). Called *transdisciplinary,* such collaboration crosses disciplinary lines and is sometimes controversial. Yet, clinical problems, particularly in those chronic persons whose conditions traverse inpatient and community settings, warrant innovative ideas that can quickly lead to practice changes.

The Quality-Caring Model advances the notion that intra- and interprofessional collaboration positively impacts health care outcomes and is a nursing responsibility. Using the caring factors in the day-to-day interactions with colleagues fosters healing environments that may contribute to improved quality of work life, enhanced clinical research, and earlier advances in patient care.

SUMMARY

Despite the importance of colleagueship between nurses and other members of the health care team, interprofessional insensitivities exist that diminish health care outcomes. Mutual consultation and agreement among nurses regarding aspects of patient care were stressed as a method for improving colleagueship. A special form of relationship among health professionals, *collaboration,* was defined and linked to caring behaviors. True collaboration through the use of the caring factors was emphasized as a nursing responsibility.

Examples of positive and negative interprofessional practice (IP) and an integrated approach to collaborative practice were presented. The perspectives of each member, when honored, nurture IP and provide a context for authentic collaboration. Contrasting examples of IP were presented to provide additional insight for authentic collaboration. Finally, transdisciplinary research was presented as an avenue to advanced patient care.

CALLS TO ACTION

Through nursing's common traditions, artifacts, language, and actions, professional nurses are already linked to each other. This exceptional bond offers a unique opportunity for nurses to generate even more advanced relationships—those that emanate from its caring base. **Appreciate** the value of nursing's shared heritage.

To attain superior patient and family health care goals, "being collaborative" is necessary. Being collaborative suggests a shared, reciprocal relationship that is focused on the common goal of improving patient outcomes. **Share** your true self with the health care team.

True collaboration, while mutual, also acknowledges the humanness of the individual partners while safeguarding the identity of the represented professionals. **Become familiar** with other health care professionals' obligations.

Reliably implementing caring interpersonal relationships— both with patients and families and with members of the health care team—is a nursing responsibility according to the Quality-Caring Model. Practicing this way contributes to positive patient outcomes, upholds each health care team member's unique contribution, and may increase work satisfaction. **Appraise** the consistency of your own interprofessional behavior.

Mutual problem solving suggests that professional nurses actively search out other health care providers to figure out together how best to help patients, to understand alternative views, and to jointly sort out clinical problems. Reaching out to health team members to actively listen, making the effort to participate with physicians on patient rounds, investigating lab results or other diagnostic tests, and energetically dialoguing about clinical issues are examples of this behavior. **Seek** out other health care professionals.

(continued)

Collaborative relationships mature when poised, well-integrated professional nurses use the caring factors in daily practice. **Choose** to implement the caring factors with health team members.

Reflective Questions/Applications for Students

1. Consider the term *horizontal violence* as it relates to professional nurses. Explain its meaning, including aggressive acts and bullying.
2. Differentiate between *colleagueship* and *collaboration*.
3. How do nurses demonstrate collaboration on your unit?
4. Explain how physician and nurse perspectives may differ in the care of specific patient populations.
5. Describe interprofessional practice.
6. How would you incorporate the patient into your interprofessional team?
7. List at least 5 ways professional nurses are connected to each other.
8. Discuss how interprofessional relationships can hinder or advance patient outcomes.

Reflective Questions/Applications for Educators

9. Examine the literature for best evidence regarding teaching and learning about interprofessional relationships.
10. Design learning experiences for undergraduate and graduate nursing students on interprofessional relationships.
11. List the collaborative research projects in which you are involved.

Reflective Questions/Applications for Nurse Leaders

12. How do you as a nurse leader deal with workplace violence?
13. Describe how staff nurses in your organization make new house staff feel welcome on their units.
14. What forums currently exist at your institution that promote nurse–physician collaborative relationships?
15. Describe specifically how the Quality-Caring Model can assist you in improving interprofessional practice at your organization.

16. In what ways does the organizational culture at your institution demonstrate support for interprofessional practice—be specific.

REFERENCES

American Hospital Association. (2008). *Hospital facts to know.* Retrieved September 8, 2008, from http://www.aha.org/aha/content/2008/pdf/08-issue-facts-to-know-.pdf

Baggs, J. G., Ryan, S., Phelps, C. E., Richeson, J. F., & Johnson, J. E. (1992). The association between interdisciplinary collaboration and patient outcomes in a medical intensive care unit. *Heart and Lung, 21*(1), 18–24.

Carter, L., Nelson, J. L., Stevers, B. A., Dukek, S. L., Pipe, T. B., & Holland, D. E. (2008). Exploring a culture of caring. *Nursing Administration Quarterly, 32*(1), 57–63.

Christmas, K. (2007). Workplace abuse: Finding solutions. *Nursing Economics, 25*(6), 365–367.

Clark, C. M. (2007). Student voices on faculty incivility in nursing education: A conceptual model. *Nursing Education Perspectives, 29*(5), 284–289.

Clark, C. M. (2008). Student perspectives on faculty incivility in nursing education. *Nursing Outlook, 56*(1), 4–8.

Duddle, M., & Boughton, M. (2007). Intraprofessional relations in nursing. *Journal of Advanced Nursing, 59*(1), 29–37.

Ehrmann, G. (2005). Managing the aggressive student. *Nurse Educator, 30*(3), 98–100.

Ferns, T., & Meerabeau, L. (2008). Verbal abuse experienced by nursing students. *Journal of Advanced Nursing, 61*(4), 431–444.

Geva, E., Barsky, A., & Westernoff, F. (2000). *Interprofessional practice with diverse populations.* Westport, CT: Green Publishing.

Grey, M., & Connolly, C. A. (2008). "Coming together, keeping together, working together": Interdisciplinary, to transdisciplinary research and nursing. *Nursing Outlook, 56*(3), 102–107.

The Kenneth B. Schwartz Center. (2007). *Schwartz Center Rounds.*® Retrieved December 19, 2007, from http://www.theschwartzcenter.org/programs/rounds_kit.html

Knaus, W. A., Draper, E. A., Wagner, D. P., & Zimmerman, J. E. (1986). An evaluation of outcome from intensive care in major medical centers. *Annals of Internal Medicine, 104*(3), 410–418.

Latham, C. L., Hogan, M., & Ringl, K. (2008). Nurses supporting nurses: Creating a mentoring program for staff nurses to improve the workforce environment. *Nursing Administration Quarterly, 32*(1), 27–39.

Lewis, S. E. (2006). Recognition of workplace bullying: A qualitative study of women targets in the public sector. *Journal of Community and Applied Social Psychology, 16*, 119–135.

Marshall, P., & Robson, R. (2005). Preventing and managing conflict: Vital pieces in the patient safety puzzle. *Healthcare Quarterly, 8*(Special Issue): 39–44.

Minnesota Nurses Association. (1999). *MNA position statement: Colleagueship in nursing practice.* Retrieved February 3, 2008, from http://nursesrev.advocateoffice.com/vertical/Sites/%7B41671038-B8D0-4277-90A9-50B10F730CBD%7D/uploads/%7BD5A197AD-12CF-4F80-8F82-88A2F9F097CD%7D.PDF

Reed, D. B., & Kidd, P. S. (2004). Collaboration between nurses and agricultural teachers to prevent adolescent agricultural injuries: The agricultural disability awareness and risk education model. *Public Health Nursing, 21*(4), 323–333.

Reeves, S., & Lewin, S. (2004). Interprofessional collaboration in the hospital: Strategies and meanings. *Journal of Health Services Research and Policy, 9,* 218–225.

Scott, J. G., Sochalski, J., & Aiken, L. (1999). Review of magnet hospital research: Findings and implications for professional nursing practice. *Journal of Nursing Administration, 29*(1), 9–19.

Shortell, S. M., Rosseau, D. M., Gillies, R. R., Devers, K. J., & Simons, T. L. (1992). Organizational assessment in intensive care units (ICU's): Construct development, reliability, and validity of the nurse–physician questionnaire. *Medical Care, 29,* 709–726.

6 Caring for Communities

In and through community lies the salvation of the world.
—M. Scott Peck

Keywords: **community, caring communities, community capacity**

THE NATURE OF COMMUNITY

As interacting beings, humans relate to each other throughout their lives in larger groups such as families, neighborhoods, places of worship, work, school, recreation, and today, online. As a member of a group, one shares a specific setting and similar characteristics with other individuals, and relationships among the members of a group are core to its sustainability. Traditionally, communities were defined as physical places or certain geographic regions where shared histories, local values, and cultural norms created a sense of belonging. However, communities can also be defined by occupation, such as a community of farmers or a retirement community. They can also be defined by a special interest, such as a community of users of a common software program. Usually, a community shares demographics, common attitudes, and values, has a known way of communicating and making decisions, and utilizes common resources. Over time, the word *community* has evolved to mean a "sense of community" or "being in community" (McMillan & Chavis,

1986). In this definition, four elements work together to create the meaning of community. They are: membership, influence, integration and fulfillment of needs, and shared emotional connections. Membership is further understood by parameters (such as language, dress, and rituals), emotional safety, a sense of belonging and identification, personal investment, and a common symbol system. To have this awareness of community, according to McMillan and Chavis (1986), one must feel empowered to have influence.

This latter definition of community has been used in the workplace to describe the network of relationships in which one is connected. In nursing, for example, professional organizations and even shared governance councils can be viewed as communities. According to Peck (1987), a true community demonstrates deep respect and authentic listening for the needs of others. He went on to say that inclusivity (accepting each other), commitment to a shared vision, and consensual decision making are hallmarks of true communities. Whatever definition one chooses to characterize communities, most include three factors: people, place, and function (Shuster & Goeppinger, 2004).

Today's traditional communities are facing tremendous pressures. Diverse members of society are residing in changing neighborhoods often without supportive extended families; they have to commute long distances to work, often in nauseating traffic. Places are evolving—earlier rural environments have become almost cosmopolitan, while services have not kept pace. Environmental issues such as poor quality air, water and sewage, climate change, and decreased energy sources are cropping up without real solutions. Functions of communities are different as jobs change and new ones replace them, sometimes resulting in lower tax revenues, school problems, crime and violence, and environmental toxins. The forces of globalization and Internet communication have disconnected local economies and fractured face-to-face contact. These stressors often lead to less engagement in community service and eventual frustration, apathy, and stagnation as community members begin to feel powerless over their changing circumstances.

For example, a rural fishing community of 1,200 people within 2.5 hours of a major city has seen a large influx of wealthier retirees. These older retirees are demanding high-quality health services, shopping and restaurant venues, and changes in how the land is used, including the building of large homes on the waterfront with fertilized lawns and water runoff. These changes have impacted the fishing industry (which is the livelihood of the local community) in terms of decreased supply and challenged the local health care services. Animated community meetings between the locals and the "come here's" have produced bad feelings, created several tax increases and enforcement of a new policy related to septic systems, and forced some local store owners to yield to the bigger chains. Unfortunately, the local fisherman do not see the value of improved services or new stores (for their community was just fine before the "come here's" arrived), so they often petition the town council to abandon plans for improved services. The overall function of this community as a fishing/farming town is changing. New people are moving in, stores and restaurants are opening, and the fish population is dwindling. This has forced the state to restrict fishing to ensure the future of the fish population. The locals are losing their livelihood, and the "come here's" are viewed as the reason. Such a situation represents a vicious circle of frustration that threatens to stagnate the local economy and spirit of this community.

Caring communities on the other hand support human capital and contribute to the welfare and development of community members (Eisler, 2007). They focus on the needs of members and work to nourish and strengthen their talents, their quality of life, and their connected relationships, ultimately tackling the problems they face. In this way, communities remain healthy with a preserved sense of shared identity.

CARING COMMUNITIES

In a provocative book titled *Reclaiming Higher Ground,* Lance Secretan (1997) reminds us that communities, whose members see the whole and give more than they take, can change not only themselves but others, including the larger world. According to Secretan, deriving meaning through work *and also through authentic community involvement* is a need of the soul.

Commitment of time and energy in true community partnership is a form of caring that is beneficial for health care professionals who often use their strengths only in the work environment. It is important to remember that the workplace is a part of the larger community and often is supported financially by it. By actively participating in the larger community, health care professionals are contributing to the health of the local population and their own personal growth.

Caring communities can take on many forms. A fundamental principle is *enabling members* through information and education, establishing linkages, and organizing and procuring resources. The key to caring communities is the network of relationships among members and the informal day-to-day exchanges that occur among them. When relationships among members of a community are of a caring nature, individuals feel safe and dignified, resulting in richer public events. Because most community involvement is voluntary, it is important that members see the value of their participation so that continued movement is possible.

One form of caring communities is the practice community. Practice communities are groups of people who engage in collective learning about a shared domain. Usually they have a particular passion for the domain and engage in joint activities to learn together how to do it better. Members are usually practitioners of some sort who build relationships with each other to further their interest in the discipline (Wenger, 1998). According to Wenger, who first coined the term *community of practice,* members of a practice community learn from each other through relationship in informal exchanges. Leading companies have used such communities to augment knowledge development and innovation (Lesser & Storck, 2001). Practice communities in health care, for example, might be formed based on redesigning patient care delivery systems, the use of a common instrument, or combining resources to achieve a cost saving. The value of cultivating such communities could be tremendous in terms of decreasing rework, increasing innovation, and increasing patient satisfaction.

Many initiatives are ongoing in health care to increase participation by providers in larger community groups. For example, one vice president for nursing in the mid-Atlantic region who understands this concept has encouraged her staff to contribute to the local community by recognizing them through specialized reward systems for their community efforts. Their contributions have led to decreased risk factors for cardiovascular disease, improved access to prenatal care, and increased adolescent knowledge about chronic diseases, all contributors to healthy communities.

Nurse educators use service-learning concepts as strategies to bridge the gap between classroom and community. One example of this is the work of Dr. Anne E. Belcher, DNS, RN, at Indiana University (Indiana University, 2006). Since the mid-1980s, Dr. Belcher has designed activities that drew her undergraduate nursing students out of the classroom and into the community where they could learn nursing in the context of helping members of the community. She established partnerships with Marion County Health Department and the Indianapolis Public Schools (IPS), the latter to teach breast and testicular self-examination to high school students. This program has now extended beyond the original five IPS high schools to township and parochial high schools throughout Marion County. In addition, she established the Indiana Childhood Immunization Outreach Program (1995–1997), a project that created partnerships between the regional campuses of the university and local public health nurses to increase their knowledge base about best immunization practices. Another exemplar is the Health Promotion Learning Cooperative, a program that partners the School of Nursing and School of Physical Education with an urban community high school to increase emphasis on exercise, nutrition, and fitness. The program provides personal physical trainers and health coaching for students, staff, and community residents. Most recently, Dr. Belcher participated in a service learning opportunity using health report cards to assess the level of health and fitness in a community, and then she designed (together with the nursing students) appropriate health education programming. These projects established genuine linkages between a school of nursing, its students, and the community that positively affected student learning and overall community health. Engaging members of the local community by offering information and education assisted nursing students to expand their knowledge of nursing and appreciation of cultural diversity by participating directly in the community in which they lived. It created linkages between a school of nursing and multiple community agencies that will be sustained by the caring relationships established by Dr. Belcher.

At the graduate level, examples of community-based nursing programs are plentiful. Recently, however, increasing focus has been placed on global and immigrant health, preparing advanced practice nurses to improve access, decrease barriers, and reduce health disparities in underserved immigrants and refugees, and improve local emergency preparedness (MastersinNursing.com, 2008).

Many nurse researchers routinely partner with community agencies to trial interventions that may enhance the health of the community. Parish nurses use caring practices within their faith communities to promote health. Connecting to the larger community in which one lives provides unique experiences that promote meaning in one's life.

BUILDING COMMUNITY CAPACITY USING
THE QUALITY-CARING MODEL©

Building community capacity refers to developing the infrastructure (ways and means) to take on the challenges of community life. Communities need this capacity to tackle their problems and to preserve their unique life ways. Without regular interaction among citizens, communities are unable to move forward, ensure social justice, build collective resilience (needed in times of disasters), and promote the common good, in other words, they become unhealthy. Healthy communities, on the other hand, demonstrate authentic citizen participation in which old and new ideas are included. Building community capacity is a civic duty to which health care providers can greatly contribute.

Using the caring factor *mutual problem solving,* nurses who participate in community groups can provide health care information, brainstorm with citizens to find solutions, explore multiple ways of dealing with community health issues, help citizens figure out questions to ask authorities, do literature searches, validate citizens' perceptions of health issues, actively listen, engage citizen groups in discussion, and facilitate group process. This factor ensures member engagement and inclusion, both necessary for healthy communities.

Being accessible and available for group meetings is important because it demonstrates commitment. The caring factor *attentive reassurance* refers to these activities and also includes a hopeful outlook for the future. In situations where citizens feel dejected or powerless, citizen nurses can use this factor to instill confidence in each other and the process. Such actions promote a sense of possibility, the antidote to despair.

Human respect, the third caring factor, is essential to promoting the sense of belonging/inclusion that citizen groups need for sustainability. Humans in community are significant members who play a part in the vibrancy of the overall community. Realizing the fundamental value of each human person as he or she contributes in community activities by recognizing their name, celebrating their uniqueness, and appreciating their service will signal to them that they matter; such feelings may facilitate longer-term participation and contribution.

Using an *encouraging manner* in community group activities provides "safe space" for citizens to enter discussions and share ideas. Such a demeanor is enthusiastic and supportive. It offers members opportunities to express their feelings even if they are negative. It is an open stance, with verbal and nonverbal congruency, that promotes support.

Nurses are experts at this factor and should use it liberally while participating in community activities.

> While individual members of communities share a common history, there are contextual differences that must be appreciated and honored if ongoing authentic participation is to endure. Using the caring factor *appreciation of unique meanings*, nurses participating in community groups can recognize members' unique frames of reference and then acknowledge and honor them through communications and actions that maintain their worldview. Nurses do this all the time in practice as they strive to see health care situations from the patient's point of view. This caring factor requires knowing individuals enough to appreciate what is important to them. When individuals sense that their worldview is honored, they feel understood and empowered.

Individuals active in community groups often meet in community-based settings that may or may not facilitate authentic discussion. Nurses can help create a *healing environment* that is private, free of stressors, safe, and aesthetically appealing by ensuring that the physical setting is clean, wheelchair accessible, has adequate and balanced lighting, fresh air/adequate ventilation, clean water, is free of hazards, and is private so that individuals are comfortable as they debate and problem solve community concerns. Going one step farther, nurses can even facilitate therapeutic surroundings through volunteering to add soft paint, works of arts, resources, and plantings. The objective is to help individuals feel welcome, balanced, and at home—in essence, a place where they belong.

Meeting *basic human needs* is a caring factor that seems out of place in community groups. Yet, how often do nurses notice unhealthy behaviors in people that weren't the reason they sought health care in the first place?

> Community participation is a great place to role model, observe, and help meet the basic needs of individuals who may otherwise not think to seek health care. For example, nurses participating in
> *(continued)*

community groups could ensure that food and beverage choices were kept healthy. They could use opportunities for health teaching about needs for sleep and relaxation and help individuals with higher-level needs through appropriate referrals. Finally, remembering that individuals have families and including them in community activities meets *affiliation needs,* an important caring factor.

Consider this example from Minnesota in which a nurse organized citizens to create a plan for decreasing teen alcohol rates.

A local newspaper reported that a statewide student health survey revealed their school district had one of the highest teen alcohol-use rates in the whole state. Numerous letters to the editors questioned why the community was not doing anything about the problem. Some viewed the report as an affront to the community's reputation (in the words of their city welcome sign) as a great place to raise children. A demand was put out for community action.

A nurse from the public health agency partnered with other community groups and organizations to develop a plan to address alcohol use in the community. The plan included recommendations for enforcing existing laws (such as tightening sales of alcohol and enforcing "not a drop" laws with minors), as well as developing acceptable (that is, "cool") alcohol-free activities for adolescents. The group's other major thrust was a decision to study assets and protective factors in adolescents to see if the community could find ways to develop assets in addition to preventing risk-taking behaviors. The representatives of each organization (including the nurse) were asked to take back this idea and get a commitment from their respective boards for the plan. (Minnesota Department of Health, 2006, p. 32)

The nurse in this example took action in her community using relationships as the basis for organizing an action plan to decrease a major public health threat. More specifically, she used mutual problem solving to brainstorm ideas, and she was available and treated her partners with respect. She allowed all points of view to be heard and helped her partners feel accepted and understood.

Another example from a judicious group of student nurses shows how a clinical problem in one setting can be the basis for a longer-term, community-based health program:

A student nurse and her colleagues noticed that a number of their postpartum clients were experiencing depression. As part of a school assignment she searched the literature for further understanding of their observations. She discovered that postpartum depression is a very serious condition that has an early onset during the first six months after birth and affects 10–20% of new mothers. In the process of reading the literature, she also learned of a screening tool that is effective in screening women for postpartum depression—the Edinburgh Postnatal Depression Scale. It takes approximately 5 minutes to administer and identifies postpartum women at high risk for depression. The students were convinced that they could improve the health status of postpartum women in their county by systematically screening for depression. They proposed that all nurses in their agency screen all postpartum women for depression using the tool and place the results in the client's record. Then, follow-up screening between 4–6 weeks postpartum at their primary care providers' offices was recommended. Referrals would be made based on written protocols. The long-range plan was to gather baseline data that demonstrates the effectiveness of screening postpartum women for depression. (Minnesota Department of Health, 2006, p. 13)

While the students were bound by their classroom activities, they showed initiative and courage in developing an evidence-based idea that could improve the health of their community. Using mutual problem solving, they searched the literature, found a practical screening tool, and proposed a solution. Following up on this idea would require education, partnerships with primary health care providers, and research skills—all dependent on high-quality relationships.

As many have speculated, most ill persons prefer to remain in their communities (versus receiving inpatient care). In fact, in one neighborhood of older adults, the citizens formed a group to discuss their health care needs. As a result of several meetings, the group admitted their desire to remain independent throughout their older years. They eventually committed to caring for each other, including making meals, doing laundry, providing transportation, and even helping with activities of daily living just to ensure they would not be hospitalized or sent to a nursing home! Nurses, as experts in caring, can greatly enhance community capacity through their authentic involvement. Using the caring factors, they can help to cultivate healthy communities—those that have certain characteristics that assist them to advance (see Table 6.1). Healthy communities are fundamental to the health and safety of their citizens. They allow citizens to have a voice, promote quality of life, economic opportunity, and raise hope for the future. In healthy communities, there is

Table 6.1

HEALTHY AND UNHEALTHY COMMUNITIES

HEALTHY	UNHEALTHY
Organic	Structured
Dynamic/Open communication	Apathetic/Closed communication
Inclusive	Narrow-minded
Connected	Isolated
Regular interactions	Infrequent interactions
Possibilities	Hopelessness
Supportive	Unhelpful
Human	Fragmented
Safe/balanced	Insecure
Empowered	Prohibitive

noticeable collaboration between private and governmental services and attractive, clean surroundings. These outcomes are of special interest to nurses who are advocates for good health. Actively engaged nurses who participate in their larger communities will not only realize great personal benefits but will ensure the ongoing vitality of the community.

SUMMARY

Human beings seem to need a sense of being part of something larger than the family—a *community.* Such a group of similar individuals is often bounded geographically or occupationally. In today's world, they can also be defined by special interests (i.e., a practice community). A "sense of community" is fostered when membership, influence, integration, fulfillment of individual needs, and emotional connections are understood and shared. Contemporary communities are undergoing unprecedented change often with negative consequences. Caring communities, on the other hand, offer rich support and can strengthen the health and quality of life among the members. Professional nurses are key to building caring communities that thrive.

CALLS TO ACTION

A group's ability to carry on is dependent on the relationships among its members. Actively **support** the members of your working group.

Lasting involvement in and commitment to community activities is facilitated by respecting the innate worth of each human person as he or she engages, calling him or her by name, honoring whatever is contributed, and recognizing their service. **Learn** more about the members of your immediate community.

Nurses who participate in community groups use the caring-factor appreciation of unique meanings by having an appreciation for each member's worldview and then using it to communicate and perform their group duties. **Join** a community group today.

Reflective Questions/Applications for Students

1. Define the term *community*.
2. Explain the elements that work together to create the meaning of community.
3. Describe the pressures facing the community in which you live and work.
4. Discuss the term *caring communities*. How is it different or the same as the word *communities?* What is its focus? Name three caring communities.
5. How does the local community support your place of employment?
6. What community groups does your organization routinely interact with?
7. Define community capacity.
8. Name the community groups in which you actively participate.
9. Consider a community group in your area. Describe their capacity. Describe how you could use the caring factors to move the group forward.

Reflective Questions/Applications for Educators

10. How do students in your program of study learn about the health problems of the surrounding community?
11. What service learning activities are ongoing at your institution? How are you involved?
12. What participatory action research studies are ongoing at your institution that include genuine community partnerships as the basis for change?

Reflective Questions/Applications for Nurse Leaders

13. What communities of practice are apparent in your organization? What domain are they organized around? Who are the members? Who are the leaders? What do they learn about?
14. Using the community in which you live, describe the major health problems encountered by its citizens. What strengths can your organization bring to help address these issues? How would you evaluate this effort?

REFERENCES

Eisler, R. (2007). *The real wealth of nations.* San Francisco, CA: Berrett-Koehler Publishers, Inc.

Indiana University. (2006). *Thomas Ehrlich Award for Excellence in Service Learning.* Retrieved May 28, 2008, from http://newsinfo.iu.edu/news/page/normal/3174.html

Lesser, E. L., & Storck, J. (2001). Communities of practice and organizational performance. *IBM Systems Journal, 40*(4), 831–841.

MastersinNursing.com. (2008). *Guide to accredited schools offering Master's degrees in nursing.* Retrieved May 16, 2008, from http://www.urlwire.com/news/060608.html

McMillan, D. W., & Chavis, D. M. (1986). Sense of community: A definition and theory. *American Journal of Community Psychology, 14*(1), 6–23.

Minnesota Department of Health. (2006). *A collection of "Getting Behind the Wheel" stories 2000–2006.* Minneapolis, MN: Office of Public Health Practice.

Peck, M. S. (1987). *The different drum: Community-making and peace.* New York: Simon and Schuster.

Secretan, L. (1997). *Reclaiming higher ground: Creating organizations that inspire the soul.* Ontario, Canada: The Secretan Center.

Shuster, G. F., & Goeppinger, J. (2004). Community as client: Assessment and analysis. In M. Stanhope & J. Lancaster (Eds.), *Community and public health nursing.* New York: Elsevier.

Wenger, E. (1998). *Communities of practice: Learning, meaning, and identity.* Cambridge, England: Cambridge University Press.

The Power of Relationships for Advancing Health Care Quality

7 Leading Quality Caring

Our chief want is someone who will inspire us to be what we know we could be.

—Ralph Waldo Emerson

Keywords: relationship-centered leadership, organizational caring

THE CONTEXT OF PROFESSIONAL NURSING PRACTICE

The current demands of the complex health care system have been associated with approximately 40% of professional nursing time spent *away* from patients and families (Krischbaum et al., 2007). In fact, a recent study of registered nurses (RNs) from 14 medical–surgical units in 3 midwestern hospitals revealed that they spent 44% of their time in direct patient care, 36% of their time in non–value added work, 7% of their time teaching, and less than 7% of their time delivering traditional psychosocial care (Storfjell, Omoike, & Ohlson, 2008). Costs were calculated for the non–value added RN work and averaged $757,000 per nursing unit annually! Labeled complexity compression by Krischbaum and her colleagues (2007), the phenomenon of nursing time spent in nondirect patient care while simultaneously performing direct patient care in a compressed time frame, is serious because professional nurses

113

are the key to patient safety and quality in hospitals. To complicate matters, Pilette (2005) has reported that many RNs "show up for work but because of mental, medical, or other personal conditions, do not function or perform at 100%" (p. 300). Labeling this *presenteeism,* a cousin of *absenteeism,* she discusses the practice of increasingly more RNs coming to work when they should not, or when employees put in excessive work hours, resulting in being physically present at work but functionally absent. To summarize the context of the professional practice environment today, RNs are struggling to provide quality patient care while supervising increasingly more unlicensed assistive personnel and juggling multiple personal and professional responsibilities. Working this way is discouraging and counter to the relationship-oriented nature of nursing. It often leads to feelings of alienation and a focus on daily operations or tasks (in order to accomplish them in a reduced time frame). In nursing, this further translates into loss of meaning in the work that has implications for job satisfaction, intent to leave, and actual resignation.

Prior research has demonstrated that the nursing practice environment is a strong predictor of job satisfaction and turnover (Irvine & Evans, 1995; Laschinger, 2008; Schmalenberg & Kramer, 2008; Ulrich, Buerhaus, Donelan, Norman, & Dittrus, 2005; Upenieks, 2003). In a more recent study of 168 Pennsylvania hospitals, Aiken, Clarke, Sloane, Lake, and Cheney (2008) found that care environments (measured as three subscales, namely staff development and quality management; nurse manager ability, leadership, and support; and collegial nurse–physician relationships) were tied to more positive nurse job experiences and lower risks of patient death and failure to rescue. Keeping this in mind, nursing leaders at all levels are faced daily with the complexity of the practice setting. Listening to and solving patient and family complaints, providing adequate staffing and supervision during a severe shortage, planning for the future, assuming financial responsibility, ensuring that patient care delivery systems meet patient needs, motivating employees, managing politics and ethical dilemmas, and ensuring positive patient outcomes using sophisticated performance improvement models dominate the leader's time. As the nursing shortage intensifies, maintaining adequate staffing is becoming a priority, with staff nurses increasingly looked upon as resources and bonus pay and flexible scheduling as recruiting incentives. This point of view may initially attract nurses, but long-term retention becomes problematic as they feel unconnected to the whole and are less likely to develop satisfying interpersonal relationships. So the unending spiral of staffing continues and consumes nursing leaders' time. As with patient care, nursing leaders are spending less and less time nurturing interprofessional caring relationships and developing the professional practice of nursing and more time recruiting new nurses. The demands of the work are overriding the time and effort it takes to build a caring professional practice environment. To make matters worse, issues of emotional overload, diversity, harassment, external forces, and controlling both human and environmental resources complicate relationship building. In essence, nursing leaders have done exactly what staff nurses have done—buried their caring nature—in what seems to be more important responsibilities. Yet, if organizations, comprised of people who live and work in relationship, are to be understood as complex living systems, the importance of relationship must emerge as a central theme. Furthermore, as primary directors of the discipline of nursing in an organization, nursing leaders are responsible for demonstrating to the organization "how expert nursing practice makes a difference to outcomes of care" (Cathcart, 2008, p. 87), ensuring success of the organization while simultaneously shaping nursing practice in a significant manner such that the professional integrity of staff nurses is maintained. To do this, nursing leaders must own and genuinely connect to the practice of nursing using caring relationships as the underlying foundation.

Dr. Marilyn Ray (1997) espoused the importance of nurse administrators' modeling caring in order to connect and create authentic relationships with staff. Such action makes caring visible and grounds decisions in a caring ethic that informs future interactions with staff and preserves the good of the organization as a whole. In 2001, Ray revised the theory of bureaucratic caring to emphasize the interconnectedness of health care institutions including the integration of caring relationships with various organizational dimensions (such as political, economic, and legal), and she offered the theory as a guide to administrative practice. Using a caring ethic as a basis for decision making and recognizing caring as having economic value, nurse leaders can positively enhance quality care.

RELATIONSHIP-CENTERED LEADERSHIP

At the core of health care organizations are the specific ways that human employees relate to each other and the organization itself. These ways of relating uniquely characterize the organization and hold a special purpose for organizational change and/or growth. Yet, they often go unnoticed and therefore untapped as resources for organizational advancement and/or renewal. In organizations that serve others, ongoing interaction and self-organization are natural. Oftentimes interactions among groups of people (or teams) are more important than the discrete actions of the individuals alone. A beneficial or generative relationship occurs when interactions among individuals of a complex system produce valuable, novel, and unconventional capabilities that are not the result of any one of them acting alone. Therefore, thinking and behaving together, or to put it differently, complex interactive whole system relating, can often maximize the potential of organizations while facilitating improved outcomes for individuals (e.g., learning, empowerment, personal development).

Seen from this perspective, continuous interactions and relationship-building form a different paradigm for leadership—one that frames it as connected, interdependent, organic, interactive, alive, creative, and whole—where the system continuously recreates itself. Moreover, the *quality* of relationships within organizations often counters the stress and uncertainty of today's complexity. In other words, how connected one feels to the organization or his/her work group determines to some extent how well he/she will share ideas, pay attention to and take responsibility for one's own practice, learn, and try new methods. Safran, Miller, and Bechman (2006) described seven relationship qualities that determine the extent to which organizations can grow, change, and thrive. They are:

Mindfulness

Diversity of mental models

Heedful interrelating

A mix of rich and lean communication

A mix of social and task-related interactions

Mutual respect

Trust

These characteristics are aligned with ideas such as self-awareness, openness, appreciating various ways of thinking and approaching decisions, creativity, attentive interactions, a combination of direct face-to-face communication together with indirect methods, honesty, valuing all human persons, security, and risk-taking behaviors, *all dimensions of caring!*

Leadership based on relationships acknowledges the interdependent nature of human beings and recognizes that change occurs naturally in complex systems and will spread more quickly if leaders attend to relationships *as the primary component of their job*. The leader's role is to cultivate a culture of inclusion, create safe space for discussion, facilitate information and knowledge, hold up professional standards, and allow others to adapt their practices in ways that are most meaningful to them. Such leadership is relationship-centered and transpersonal. It sees the human person in the employee and, in this case, the inherent caring nature of nurses. Relationship-centered leadership honors and preserves the special relationship that nurses have with patients and families.

As Sumner and Townsend-Rocchiccioli (2003) put it, "there must be an appreciation of the unique very human relationship between nurse and patient . . . that inspired nurses to feel confident about their special contribution to positive patient outcomes" (p. 171). Ensuring that nurses experience the full and deep meaning of nursing with its resultant opportunities for personal growth instills enthusiasm and zeal about the profession that preserves its soul and creates a practice environment of joy and gratitude. Real connection to the individuals they serve along with autonomy and self-expression enables one to relax, feel safe, and commit to quality practice. Such a compelling mission provides the motivation for nurses to work productively and stay employed. Nurse leaders who embrace the caring relationships nurses have with patients and families understand and work hard to preserve them; after all, these relationships provide the life lessons and renewal that inspire staff nurses to continue their important work!

Transpersonal or relationship-centered leaders lead from within; that is, they halt the "thinking and doing" mode often enough to reflect, enter sacred space, become aware, and cultivate the self (see chapter 3). Caring leadership, as executive practice, requires the capacity to care for self. Koloroutis (2002) listed the attributes of caring leaders. They are:

Emotionally present

Able to see beyond current problems/situations

Possess positive energy

Have a hope-filled attitude, consistently seeing possibilities

Honest, truth telling even when it is difficult

Open, good listeners, seeking to understand

Respectful; believing in others

Supportive and encouraging

And while not listed as an attribute, physical health, including diet and exercise and adequate sleep, is a prerequisite for attentive and focused behavior, while reflective and expressive practices add depth to relationships that is healing. Borchardt (2002) asserts that nurse leaders have a responsibility to model healthy lifestyles. Nurse leaders at all levels need time for renewal to continuously remain in relationship-mode.

Executive nurse leaders stimulate a culture of caring in an organization and maintain the focus on caring relationships that demonstrates its high priority. Creating unity of purpose, setting high expectations, and consistently reminding employees why they are there influence positive interactions that fuel advancement. In a relationship-centered context, executive leaders' work "shifts naturally from producing results to encouraging the growth of people who produce results" (Senge, Scharmer, Jaworski, & Flowers, 2004, p. 141). In fact, in Senge and colleagues' *Presence,* the chapter on leadership is titled "Leadership: Becoming a Human Being" (p. 177). Even during conflict, staying "in relationship" through continued dialogue leads to a deeper connection that over time may bring about resolution of the conflict. A transpersonal leader is able to synthesize caring relationships and the bottom line by what Bill Torbert (2004) called *action inquiry.* Reflective listening followed by appropriate action—being *both* in action and inquiry at the same time—requires an integrated individual who knows him/herself in relation to others. This open stance temporarily suspends action; it notices and then acts through caring relationships to advance the system. It requires leaders to have confidence in the organization's wisdom or belief in its people. Techniques such as appreciative inquiry that use positive, hopeful, and engaging methods to promote organizational change or partnerships serve to "appreciate" the strengths of a system and use them in innovative ways (Havens, Wood, & Leeman, 2006; Sherwood, 2006). Margaret Wheatley (2005) reminds us, "the primary task of being a leader is to make sure that the organization knows itself" (p. 69), while a "critical task is to increase the number, variety and strength of connections within the system" (p. 93).

Unit-level leaders are pivotal to the success of relationship-centered caring. They set the tone of a department and through visible, hands-on leadership look for and encourage the small changes that individuals make. Through the constant focus on the centrality of caring to patient outcomes, unit-level leaders encourage staff to contribute; over time, more individuals interact and become engaged, leading to larger changes. The unit-level leader who is self-aware encourages others to practice and develop their own mindfulness practices. He/she brings staff members together, keeps them informed, and helps them learn about relationships while simultaneously encouraging them to innovate. (See Table 7.1 for a description of the roles of nurse executives and unit-level nurse leaders.)

An example of such leadership occurred in a midsized community hospital during implementation of a professional practice model. The unit-level leader met each morning at 7:30 with the day and night staff together to "de-brief" about components of the model, discuss any issues or concerns regarding implementation, and provide education and encouragement. She did this *everyday for 3 months* during the pilot period. In addition, she frequently could be found in patient rooms seeking their feedback and often recognized those nurses publicly who were able to integrate the model into their daily practice. Among the four units who participated, this unit performed most effectively; the staff attributed their success to the leadership of their unit leader.

Empirical research demonstrates significant linkages between clinician–patient relationship quality and health care outcomes such as

Table 7.1

NURSE EXECUTIVES AND UNIT-LEVEL RELATIONSHIP-CENTERED LEADERSHIP ROLES

NURSE EXECUTIVE	UNIT-LEVEL LEADERSHIP
Maintain unity of purpose—quality caring	Set tone for departmental relationships
Stimulate constant learning	Visible, hands-on
Set high expectations	Recognize and reward quality caring
Maintain open stance	Bring individuals together
Provide support	Recognize and celebrate small changes
Practice self-awareness	Practice self-awareness

patient adherence (DiMatteo, 1994), symptom relief (Stewart, Brown, & Donner, 2000), satisfaction (Dingman, Williams, Fosbinder, & Warnnick, 1999; Duffy, 1992; Wolf, Colahan, & Costell, 1998; Yeakel, Maljanian, Bohannon, & Couloumbe, 2003), postoperative recovery (Swan, 1998), and positive emotional outcomes such as mood and self-esteem (Swanson, 1999). Such evidence obliges nursing leaders to pay attention to this untapped potential and promote relationships as the foundation of organizational work. Seen in this fashion, the traditional roles of management (including staffing) are allowed to occur naturally rather than artificially imposing or allocating them. Attending to the business of cultivating and sustaining caring relationships becomes the primary role of leadership.

BUILDING CAPACITY FOR ORGANIZATIONAL CARING

Although many traditional management functions are eased when relationships become the priority of leadership, facilitating an infrastructure that supports them is paramount. Two dually balanced arrangements, a patient care delivery system and a shared leadership structure, help to ensure caring professional practice and a passionate and caring nursing workforce. To that end, the Quality-Caring Model© can provide the foundation for organizing a relationship-centered patient care delivery system that honors the holistic nature of humans (Duffy & Hoskins, 2003). Using a nursing model to design how work is accomplished also changes how decisions are made (see Table 7.2).

Because the model views independent and collaborative relationships as the primary responsibility of professional nurses, maximizing time "in relationship" is a guiding principle. Other tenets drawn from the model that can offer direction include:

Patients and families are entitled to caring relationships with nurses.

Patients and families should interact with a limited number of people while hospitalized so that depth of relationship can be nurtured.

The patient–nurse relationship informs practice—the core of nursing work is caring.

Time spent interacting is expected, valued, and rewarded.

As knowledge workers, professional nurses must be able to access, critically appraise, and appropriately use the professional literature.

Table 7.2

CHANGING CHARACTERISTICS OF DECISION MAKING USING A PROFESSIONAL PRACTICE MODEL AS A FOUNDATION FOR PRACTICE

PRACTICE	LEADERSHIP	COMMENTS/IMPLICATIONS
Nursing values provide the foundation for practice	A body of nursing knowledge together with sound administrative principles provides the foundation for decision making	Leaders facilitate nursing values by their actions
RN control over practice decisions (autonomy)	Less dependence on leadership/advanced practitioners for decision making at the bedside; leaders are facilitators of the model	Requires critical reasoning skills; expectations of RN accountability and advocacy for high-quality nursing practice
Emphasis on improved nursing-sensitive patient outcomes	Expectation and support for RN active participation in QI/EBP/PBE	Knowledge of principles of QI/research
RNs have meaningful impact on system decisions	RNs, through shared leadership activities, contribute to system decisions	RN participation is expected, input is valued and used by leadership
Model drives the patient care and RN work environment	Structural changes may be needed to support nursing practice	Example: lighting, artwork, timing of activities
Improved image and enhanced RN job satisfaction	Less day-to-day clinical decisions; more mutual decision making	Expertise in the caring factors is needed

Collaborative relationships with the health care team inform practice—they are not optional.

Responsibility for cultivating and sustaining a caring-healing-protective environment rests on all.

Using these guiding principles, nursing leadership can work together with staff nurses to craft an innovative patient care delivery system that "honors the vital role of nursing while responding to the unique needs of patients and families" (Duffy, Baldwin, & Mastorovich, 2007, p. 547). An example of such a system can be found in Figure 7.1.

In this model, developed jointly among staff, leaders, and a faculty researcher using principles of whole system change (Bunker & Alban, 1996), the work of professional nurses was delineated as relationship-centered, and some nonrelational tasks were delegated to assistive personnel. A resource coordinator was used to reduce non–value added work such as supply procurement, an aesthetically pleasing environment, and working equipment. Registered nurses in this model were accountable for intent, competence, and autonomous practice and participated in shared leadership councils. Nursing assistants (NAs) were assigned to RNs in an 80:20 staffing ratio (80% RNs and 20% NAs) based on the available evidence (Aiken et al., 2002). Nursing assistants were valued for their contributions to patient care and offered ongoing on-site continuing education (in the event professional nursing was their career goal).

Scheduling in this system was accomplished via a self-scheduled computerized system where RNs who chose 12-hour shifts were required to work at least two consecutive days/nights, and RNs who chose

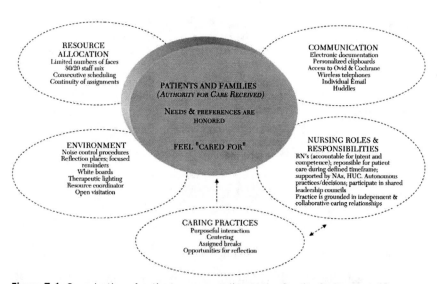

Figure 7.1 Organization of patient care according to the Quality-Caring Model.©
RN = registered nurse; NA = nursing assistant; HUC = health unit coordinator.

From "Using the Quality-Caring Model to Organize Patient Care Delivery," by J. Duffy, J. Baldwin, and M. J. Mastorovich, 2007, *Journal of Nursing Administration, 37*(12), 546–551.

8-hour shifts were required to work at least three consecutive days/ nights. Four-hour shifts were not routinely scheduled, and continuity of assignments was the rule. Such scheduling ensured that patients could interact with fewer nurses and effectively establish caring relationships. Registered nurses carried wireless telephones and clipboards with the Situation-Background-Assessment-Recommendation (SBAR) inscribed on them to ensure effective and efficient communication (Hohenhaus, Powell, & Hohenhaus, 2006). In addition, RNs had individual e-mail and access to electronic databases. They also were taught the value of the "huddle" for immediate resolution of system problems (such as several admissions at once) or conflict resolution (Institute for Healthcare Improvement, 2008).

In this patient care delivery system, caring practices or specific actions that maximized RN interaction with patients and families were developed and implemented. For example, purposeful interaction—five minutes of dedicated, uninterrupted time spent with patients—was instituted on all shifts. Building this small amount of time into the staffing pattern allowed RNs to mutually get to know their patients and fostered the notion of ongoing engagement. Centering practices and opportunities for reflection were also built into the practice culture to distinguish the nursing units as places of openness and inclusion and to create a "caring milieu within which to work and heal" (Duffy et al., 2007, p. 549). White boards installed in each patient room with the questions: What do you want to be called while in the hospital? What do you do when you are not in the hospital? and What is most important to you? were answered on admission to encourage all those who entered to come to know the patient as a person. After one year of implementation, patient satisfaction, patient-reported pain, nurse vacancy rates, and nurse satisfaction improved. Two years later, patient-reported pain and patient satisfaction continue to improve while pressure ulcer rates, patient falls, and medication errors have decreased.

Just as a patient care delivery system forms the infrastructure for caring professional practice, a shared leadership system, or governance model is necessary for today's decision-making. Because nurse work is knowledge work, RNs increasingly have more information to share, desire input, and want to make an impact on health care organizations. "Shared leadership occurs when all members of a team are fully engaged in the leadership of the team and are not hesitant to influence and guide their fellow team members in an effort to maximize the potential of the team as a whole" (Pearce, 2004, p. 48). This definition connotes mutuality, equality, inclusion, and comfort between staff and leadership whereby both perspectives are acknowledged and decisions are made jointly *in the best interest of the patient.* Groups of RNs organized around key dimensions (such as practice, education, research), typically called councils, can have great influence on the success of a nursing department. Designing these teams, including the purpose, resources, membership, and procedures, along with facilitating the boundaries of the teams, is the role of leadership (Pearce, 2004). Using caring relationships as the basis for design and facilitation of teams stimulates systems' thinking, engagement, creative thinking, and empowerment. It ensures preservation of human dignity and maximizes motivation and, ultimately, success. Likewise, establishing alliances with community partners, schools of nursing, and others can be best served by caring relationships.

USING THE QUALITY-CARING MODEL TO LEAD

The two relationships necessary for effective nursing leadership are those with staff nurses and those with other leaders in the organization. Holding these relationships close and actively working to strengthen them through inclusion and connection—essentially, hardwiring caring—is the secret to small changes that eventually allow large transformational change to emerge. While the caring factors are most often applied in direct patient care (see chapter 2), they can also serve as guides for administrative nursing practice as the foundation for words and actions, writing (including e-mail), and decision making. For example, *mutual problem solving* is a behavior that helps staff nurses make decisions and solve problems in a manner acceptable to themselves and administration. As leaders provide information, help staff see the bigger picture (whole system thinking), explore alternatives, brainstorm together, and validate perceptions, they provide a safe atmosphere for planning a course of action. Leaders who accept feedback from staff and use it to make decisions convey caring. Implicit in performing this way is comfort "in relationship"; an open, engaging stance and reciprocal, shared dialogue. An example of this caring factor can be found during discussions about staffing or lack of resources after a sick call. As staff nurses convey their displeasure about working "short," the caring nurse leader will listen, then take the time to explain the budgeted staffing pattern and how the organization is paying the nurse who is sick despite the fact that he/she is not physically at work. Adding another staff member to cover this position temporarily increases the budget and puts the unit "at variance." Once understood, the leader could invite the remaining staff to come up with alternatives—call in another nurse today and work short another day, call in another nurse today and allow staff to take vacation during downtime later in the month, or remain as is. With the staff mutually making the decision with the nurse leader, not only is the budget upheld, but nurses feel part of the solution and may be better able to understand the relationship of absenteeism and the budget.

Attentive reassurance—being physically present often with an optimistic outlook—is nurturing to staff and conveys the leader's recognition of them. Noticing and listening to staff, acknowledging changes or improvements and their caring behaviors, or a gentle affirmative touch shows nurses that they matter and builds confidence in the system. Using appropriate humor to lighten stressful situations and taking the time to appreciate someone's effort can be transforming. Of course, practicing this caring factor requires frequent interaction with staff, so rounding, assistance with certain activities, or joint projects can provide the means to enact this factor.

Human respect conveys the worth of the unique person who is a staff nurse. Not only does it signify value for the person, but in this case, it creates an appreciation for the professional nature of the nurse. Remembering and calling the nurse by name and conversing about appropriate personal issues (such as children's sports, birthday celebrations, or marriages) can remind the staff nurse that he/she has inherent worth and is valuable to the organization.

Using an *encouraging manner* when interacting both verbally and nonverbally provides support for staff nurses that can lead to empowerment and risk-taking. Pointing out the good along with the challenging behaviors, especially during formal disciplining, helps others learn and advance in their roles. For nurses who take risks on behalf of patients or the organization, formal recognition is appropriate. For those who offer to chair a council or lead a meeting, being there with them especially for the first meeting promotes the confidence required to volunteer the next time. An example of this factor occurs when a nurse who has never written an abstract or proposal for a professional conference volunteers to do it but stipulates that he/she has never done it before. Supporting them through the writing process, artfully critiquing their work, and offering praise where appropriate are supportive behaviors that encourage the nurse to finish the task.

Appreciating the context of the staff nurse recognizes the importance of culture, past experiences, and other unique meanings that impact the work life of the nurse. Attuning to these meanings and allowing them to influence decisions at times are affirming for the individual. For example, a nurse from a different culture might be allowed to explain the origin of a certain nursing action that is pertinent to his/her culture. Followed by discussion and a search of the literature, this action might be adopted for use, upholding this individual's personal worldview.

Facilitating a *healing environment* is one of the most important leadership roles that may be tied to RN job satisfaction and patient outcomes. Such an environment includes the surroundings in which nurses work, including their privacy and safety. It also includes the organizational culture or the norms and behaviors that characterize a nursing department. Relationship-centered cultures enhance one's sense of worth and encourage one to take risks. They focus on frequent interaction, open communication, and flexibility.

Making sure that the body, mind, and spirit are in optimal condition for patient care is a role of the leader that often is tied to resources. Yet, a healthy work environment includes regular periods of relaxation, available and healthy food choices, special quiet places for reflection and renewal, and uplifting continuing education. The leader who is focused on a caring-healing-protective environment will arrange the resources to support these activities. In one hospital, the Vice President for Nursing arranged for "tea carts" where various types of teas are served during the afternoon, later in the evening, and on the night shift. This gesture has become a source of relaxation and renewal to the busy nurses who often don't take the time for such self-caring. The frequent closure of hospital cafeterias on the night shift is an example of nursing leadership not focused on the important need of night nurses for nourishing food. Often night shift employees must resort to "ordering out" or eating from the vending machines. These are poor choices for health care practitioners who teach good diet to their patients. Other examples of healing environments include the many quiet rooms or peaceful artwork that now can be found in health care organizations as well as professional continuing education focused on relaxation and mindfulness practices.

Attending to *basic human needs,* such as those described above, but also to those higher-level needs for group activities and self-esteem keeps us connected to one another and generates the confidence so necessary for safe, effective practice. *Affiliation needs* recognize and honor the extended family of the staff nurse and include them in celebrations and other work initiatives. Their special needs can also be noticed in scheduling practices.

To sum up, leadership practice is augmented by caring relationships.

> Leaders who live the caring factors use the unique network of relationships that define an organization to energize staff and other leaders by integrating the professional practice of nursing with the mission of the organization. Helping to develop caring knowledge, behaviors, and attitudes and making decisions based on a caring ethic/philosophy are responsibilities of nursing leaders. Working this way cultivates a caring-healing-protective environment that sustains passion for the work and expert care to the vulnerable persons who deserve safe and quality health care.

SUMMARY

The complexities of the modern health care system have rendered professional nursing discouraged and deficient of meaning. Caring relationships so central to expert nursing practice are buried by nursing leaders as staffing pressures and other external forces have mounted. Yet, several experts have suggested that administrative caring should ground decisions and be tapped as resources for change. Leadership based on caring relationships acknowledges the connections among humans and upholds the special relationship nurses have with patients and families. In fact, caring leaders set the tone for nursing, generate confidence in their staff, and shape the infrastructure that supports them. Use of the caring factors personally and with others energizes organizations and their employees to compete and deliver expert health care.

CALLS TO ACTION

Organizations, comprised of people who live and work in relationship, are living systems that are complex and nonlinear. Sustaining quality relationships energizes the system and influences its ability to care for itself. **Visit** http://www.plexusinstitute.org

(continued)

Protecting the caring relationships that professional nurses cultivate with patients and families is a responsibility of nurse leaders. At the end of the day, it is the patient–nurse caring relationship that provides the inspiration that drives staff nurses to continue their important work! **Safeguard** patient–nurse relationships.

A caring-based patient care delivery system together with a shared leadership structure is necessary to operationalize caring professional practice. **Review** the patient care delivery system and shared leadership structures at your organization.

Living the caring factors enables nurse leaders to make better use of the unique network of relationships that define an organization. This critical mass of relationships invigorates staff and other leaders to embrace change and aligns the professional practice of nursing with the mission of the organization. **Cultivate** caring relationships with members of your organization.

Reflective Questions/Applications for Students

1. Describe the term *presenteeism.* Do you see this phenomenon at your organization? How often? How does it relate to absenteeism? Productivity?
2. Discuss the term *knowledge work* or *knowledge worker.* What does it mean? How do professional nurses fulfill the definition of this concept?
3. Evaluate the recruiting and retention policies for professional nurses at your institution. Find the latest nurse retention data and assess how the policies are working.
4. Discuss a group interaction that was generative in nature. Who was there? What roles did the members play? How often did it meet? What were the outcomes?
5. Define each of Safran et al.'s (2006) relationship qualities.
6. How do you come to know the patient as person?
7. Explain relationship-centered leadership.
8. Complete a review of literature on the linkage between patient–nurse relationships and patient outcomes. Summarize your findings and present to your classmates.

Reflective Questions/Applications for Educators

9. Design a case study around the concept of relationship-centered leadership.

10. Critique the Guiding Principles derived from the Quality-Caring Model that direct patient care delivery systems. Offer some of your own.

11. What teaching/learning strategies do you think will best guide graduate students to apply the caring factors to leadership practice?

Reflective Questions/Applications for Nurse Leaders

12. As a leader of a caring profession, relate how you care for yourself. How do you relieve/cope with job stress? Who can you point to that listens to your concerns about work-related matters? When was the last time you enjoyed an evening out with friends? What practices do you routinely perform to help you feel a sense of harmony with yourself and your work life? How do you care for your body? Mind? Spirit?

13. Examine your calendar for the past month. Where did you spend most of your work time? What does this say about what you value?

14. Create a calendar for self-care that includes time for physical, reflective, and expressive practices. Be specific including dates, times, frequency. Now DO IT!

15. Describe a tense situation between employee/s and leadership. Explain how appreciative inquiry could have been used to ease the situation.

16. Think about the patient care delivery system at your institution. Is it relationship-based? Is caring for self and others a predominant theme? Using the Quality-Caring Model, design a patient care delivery system that fits with the organization's mission and addresses RN roles and responsibilities (what will they be held responsible and accountable for?), resources (what staffing, scheduling is necessary?), communication (how will RNs communicate with each other and the health care team?), and the environment (what is necessary to create a caring-healing-protective practice setting for patients and staff?).

17. Draw a diagram depicting the congruence between the Quality-Caring Model and the patient care delivery system developed in Number 16.

18. Discuss approximately how much time nurses spend "in relationship" at your organization. What activities do nurses perform that interfere with time spent "in relationship"? Offer some innovative ways to eliminate or decrease these activities so more time can be spent "in relationship" with patients and families.

19. Explain the approach of nursing leadership to professional nursing care at your institution. What is their involvement? How do they ensure nursing care is performed in accordance with professional standards?

20. How does shared leadership promote "what's best for the patient" at your institution?

REFERENCES

Aiken, L., Clarke, S., Sloane, D., Lake, E., & Cheney, T. (2008). Effects of hospital care environment on patient mortality and nurse outcomes. *Journal of Nursing Administration, 38*(5), 223–229.

Aiken, L. H., Clarke, S. P., Sloane, D. M., Sochalski, J., & Silber, J. H. (2002). Hospital nurse staffing and patient mortality, nurse burnout, and job dissatisfaction. *Journal of the American Medical Association, 288*, 1987–1993.

Borchardt, G. L. (2002). Said another way: Role models for health promotion: The challenge for nurses. *Nursing Forum, 35*(3), 29–32.

Bunker, B. B., & Alban, B. (1996). *Large group interventions: Engaging the whole system.* Hoboken, NJ: Wiley Publishers.

Cathcart, E. B. (2008). The role of the chief nursing officer in leading the practice: Lessons from the Benner tradition. *Journal of Nursing Administration, 32*(2), 87–91.

DiMatteo, M. R. (1994). Enhancing patient adherence to medical recommendations. *Journal of the American Medical Association, 271*, 79–83.

Dingman, S., Williams, M., Fosbinder, D., & Warnnick, J. (1999). Implementing a caring model to improve patient satisfaction. *Journal of Nursing Administration, 29*(12), 30–37.

Duffy, J. (1992). The impact of nurse caring on patient outcomes. In D. Gaut (Ed.), *The presence of caring in nursing.* New York: National League for Nursing Press.

Duffy, J. R., Baldwin, J., & Mastorovich, M. J. (2007). Using the Quality-Caring Model to organize patient care delivery. *Journal of Nursing Administration, 37*(12), 546–551.

Duffy, J. R., & Hoskins, L. M. (2003). The Quality-Caring Model©: Blending dual paradigms. *Advances in Nursing Science, 26*(1), 77–88.

Havens, D., Wood, S. O., & Leeman, J. (2006). Improving nursing practice and patient care: Building capacity with appreciative inquiry. *Journal of Nursing Administration, 36*(10), 463–470.

Hohenhaus, S., Powell, S., & Hohenhaus, J. (2006). Enhancing patient safety during hand-offs: Standardized communication and teamwork using the SBAR method. *American Journal of Nursing, 34*(7), 34–38.

Institute for Healthcare Improvement. (2008). *Use regular huddles and staff meetings to plan production and to optimize team communication.* Retrieved January 13, 2008, from http://www.ihi.org/IHI/Topics/OfficePractices/Access/Changes/Individual Changes/UseRegularHuddlesandStaffMeetingstoPlanProductionandtoOptimize TeamCommunication.htm

Irvine, D. M., & Evans, M. G. (1995). Job satisfaction and turnover among nurses: Integrating research findings across studies. *Nursing Research, 44*(4), 246–253.

Koloroutis, M. (2002). *Relationship-based care: A model for transforming practice.* Minneapolis, MN: Creative Healthcare Management.

Krischbaum, K., Diemert, C., Jacox, L., Jones, A., Koenig, P., Mueller, C., et al. (2007). Complexity compression: Nurses under fire. *Nursing Forum, 42*(2), 86–94.

Laschinger, H. K. S. (2008, April 21). Effect of empowerment on professional practice environments, work satisfaction, and patient care quality: Further testing the nursing worklife model. *Journal of Nursing Care Quality.* (Epub ahead of print.) Retrieved March 2, 2008, from http://www.jncqjournal.com/pt/re/jncq/abstract.00001786-900000000-99994.htm;jsessionid=LGLSQpV6V3K5p0PGTvtKFn1QnthJl1vlyVV0qJ pnfxxD89Z0BHW8!-1101774500!181195629!8091!-1?index=1&database=ppvovft& results=1&count=10&searchid=1&nav=search

Pearce, C. L. (2004). The future of leadership: Combining vertical and shared leadership to transform knowledge work. *Academy of Management Executives, 18*(1), 47–57.

Pilette, P. C. (2005). Presenteeism in nursing: A clear and present danger to productivity. *Journal of Nursing Administration, 35*(6), 300–303.

Ray, M. (1997). The ethical theory of existential authenticity: The lived experience of the art of caring in nursing administration. *Canadian Journal of Nursing Research, 29*(1), 111–126.

Ray, M. (2001). The theory of bureaucratic caring. In M. Parker (Ed.), *Nursing theories and nursing practice.* Philadelphia, PA: FA Davis.

Safran, D. G., Miller, W., & Bechman, H. (2006). Organizational dimensions of relationship-centered care. *Journal of General Internal Medicine, 21*(S1), S9–S15.

Schmalenberg, C., & Kramer, M. (2008). Essentials of a productive nurse work environment. *Nursing Research, 57*(1), 2–13.

Senge, P., Scharmer, O., Jaworski, J., & Flowers, B. S. (2004). *Presence. Human purpose and the field of the future.* Cambridge, MA: Society for Organizational Learning.

Sherwood, G. (2006). Appreciative leadership: Building customer-driven partnerships. *Journal of Nursing Administration, 36*(12), 551–557.

Stewart, M., Brown, J. B., & Donner, A. (2000). The impact of patient-centered care on outcomes. *Journal of Family Practice, 49*, 796–804.

Storfjell, J. L., Omoike, O., & Ohlson, S. (2008). The balancing act: Patient care time versus cost. *Journal of Nursing Administration, 38*(5), 244–249.

Sumner, J., & Towsend-Rocchiccioli, J. (2003). Why nurses are leaving nursing? *Nursing Administration Quarterly, 27*(2), 164–171.

Swan, B. A. (1998). Postoperative nursing care contributions to symptom distress and functional status after ambulatory surgery. *MEDSURG Nursing, 7*, 148–158.

Swanson, K. M. (1999). Research-based practice with women who have had miscarriages. *Image, 31*(4), 339–345.

Torbert, W. (2004). *Action inquiry: The secret of timely and transforming action.* San Francisco, CA: Berrett-Koehler Publishers, Inc.

Ulrich, B. T., Buerhaus, P. I., Donelan, K., Norman, L., & Dittrus, R. (2005). How RNs view the work environment: Results of a national survey of registered nurses. *Journal of Nursing Administration, 35*(9), 389–396.

Upenieks, V. V. (2003). The interrelationship of organizational characteristics of magnet hospitals, nursing leadership, and nursing job satisfaction. *Health Care Management, 22*(2), 83–89.

Wheatley, M. J. (2005). *Finding our way: Leadership for an uncertain time.* San Francisco, CA: Berrett-Koehler Publishers, Inc.

Wolf, Z. R., Colahan, M., & Costell, A. (1998). Relationship between nurse caring and patient satisfaction. *MEDSURG Nursing, 7*(2), 99–105.

Yeakel, S., Maljanian, R., Bohannon, R., & Couloumbe, K. (2003). Nurse caring behaviors and patient satisfaction: Improvement after a multifaceted staff intervention. *Journal of Nursing Administration, 33*(9), 434–436.

8

Teaching and Learning Quality Caring

The purpose of learning is growth, and our minds, unlike our bodies, can continue growing as we continue to live.

—Mortimer Adler

Keywords: learning, teaching, caring, pedagogy, caring competency, educational program evaluation

NURSING AS PERFORMANCE

Nursing is founded on a set of beliefs about persons, health, environments, and the social responsibilities of the nurse (American Nurses Association, 2003; Fawcett, 1984). As a practice discipline, it includes specialized knowledge and skills that ultimately converge in the clinical setting with professional actions or behaviors that contribute to the health of individuals and groups. This union of knowledge, skills, and professional behaviors is much like a performing art, similar to playing the piano. Music theory must be understood, psychomotor exercises with scales and chords are repetitively carried out to perfect the practitioner's technique, and musical pieces are rehearsed over and over again, culminating in a beautiful performance. The value of music as a social good by the musician underlies his/her performance. Nursing practice is similar. It has discipline-specific knowledge that must be comprehended and psychomotor techniques that must be perfected, and it is under-girded by an ethic of caring. It is dynamic and contextual, demanding an awareness of the self, others, and the larger systems in which it is performed. Good nursing practice requires an inquisitive nature that slowly and continuously reflects upon questions such as: What am I observing about this patient and family? What am I learning about me? What am I learning about nursing? Listening for answers to these questions over time helps one to discern what is relevant or salient about clinical situations and respond accordingly.

Yet, today's prelicensure nursing students are pressured to perform at increasingly difficult levels in shorter periods of time compared to their counterparts in the social sciences, the arts, or business. Not only does entry and continued stay in a nursing program depend on mean grades above 3.0, but athletic and other extracurricular activities are often compromised by the time constraints of clinical courses. At the graduate level, most students are working (many full time) while supporting families. As an observer in a school of nursing, one would find many students coming and going at all hours, busily working on projects, studying in the library, departing and arriving home from clinical agencies, in the classroom, working online, talking on the phone, or delivering and receiving text messages. There is little downtime or group activities, and often, classroom activities continue to be conducted in teacher-driven lecture format without many opportunities for real connection.

Building on this theme, faculty are also living demanding work lives, often running from meeting to classroom to clinical site. The nursing faculty shortage, associated low salaries, and increased emphasis on extramural funding have placed further burdens on nursing faculty that limit time spent with students (Yordy, 2006). Student–teacher relationships are compromised by the hectic lives of faculty members and their students, yet positive learning outcomes have been linked to the quality of the nursing student–teacher relationship (Gramling & Nugent, 1998; Pullen, Murray, & McGee, 2001). In fact, sustaining caring relationships with nursing students may be considered a moral responsibility of nurse educators so that caring interactions as the basis for professional practice can be instilled in graduates.

As the essence of nursing (Watson, 1979), caring and its associated attitudes and behaviors are considered a major component of professional nursing education. Since the late 1980s and early 1990s curriculum revolution (Bevis & Watson, 1989; Tanner, 1990), nurse educators have been challenged to focus more on caring relationships and inter-personal processes and less on specific content. Cook and Cullen (2003) see a crucial role for nursing educators to teach the importance of caring to counter the increasing demands on practicing nurses who have shifted their focus away from caring. Many schools of nursing integrate caring concepts into the curriculum, and some have instituted separate courses on relationship-oriented aspects of nursing. However, there remains lit-tle evidence of increased caring capacity of nursing graduates. And some students report that nursing faculty "struggle to enact the same caring behaviors they advocate" (McGregor, 2005, p. 90). For example, in a Taiwanese study of two nursing schools, the largest difference reported in students' (N = 214) perceptions of effective and ineffective clinical instructors was in interpersonal relationships (t = 30.38; p < .000; Tang, Chou, & Chiang, 2005). Another report highlighted that uncaring fac-ulty members can even hinder students' success (Poormann, Webb, & Mastorovich, 2002).

In Beck's (2001) metasynthesis of caring within schools of nurs-ing, 14 qualitative studies in schools of nursing were analyzed. Using a meta-ethnographic method, four major themes emerged: caring among faculty, faculty–nursing student caring, caring among nursing students, and caring between nursing students and patients. The central compo-nent of these themes was "reciprocal connecting," which consisted of presencing, supporting, sharing, competence, and uplifting effects. This inductive approach implied that experiencing caring in the educational environment is contagious and even has a "trickle down effect" that can be translated into the practice environment (p. 108). As suggested by Inui (2003), students in the health professions learn from the informal or hidden curriculum (what they see us do). In other words, professional caring may be best learned through the caring relationships and role modeling that faculty enact during the educational process.

LEARNING NURSING IN THE CONTEXT OF CARING RELATIONSHIPS

Teaching is more than imparting knowledge; it also is about open-ness, connection, and creativity. These last three adjectives suggest that objective (outer) as well as subjective (inner) factors are involved. Learning is traditionally the goal of formal education and, in the health professions, is a requirement for continued practice. Because nursing is a practice discipline that requires a certain level of competence, learning nursing is a lifelong process that is both contextual and developmental (Leach, 2002). According to Wheatley (2005), "knowledge is created in relationship, inside thinking, reflecting human beings" (p. 149). The student's ability to perform, therefore, is influenced by the situation (setting, teacher, patient, etc.) and is augmented by relational activities that stimulate how one is assimilating new knowledge. Reflection, that is, examining one's experiences and connecting with one's feelings, is considered a hallmark of understanding a professional practice (Schon, 1987).

> Learning nursing, then, is a continual process of acquiring knowledge externally (from professors, reading and studying literary sources, peers, other nurses in the practice setting, and research) and reflecting on that knowledge to better understand how it can be applied in a professional manner in real clinical situations.

The experiences of merging information gained from external situations together with internal reflection are dependent on relationships— with each other, the larger system, and with the self. Learning occurs best when the teacher does more than convey seemingly disconnected facts while students passively receive them. Encouraging active learning through participative approaches or using pedagogies of engagement encourages meaningful learning (Edgerton, 2001). Faculty members who design and facilitate active learning experiences in the context of relationships assist nursing students to understand complex phenomena that are connected to a larger whole, are adjusted to the situation, and are transferable to a variety of nursing situations. Such learning is better known as integrative learning (Huber, Hutchings, Gale, Breen, & Miller, 2007); it helps students synthesize separate ideas, identify patterns, and develop habits that are situation-specific. Integrative learning is being fostered nationally by the Association of American Colleges and Universities (AAC & U) as faculty members strengthen connections among various content areas.

Central to these ideas of learning is the focus on connecting to the student through relationship. Traditionally in nursing education, faculty members delivered information and then expected adequate performance on tests or rational explanations for actions during clinical experiences. The relationship between teacher and student was somewhat intimidating because the teacher was considered the expert while the student was dependent on the teacher for information and evaluation. Conversely, relationships characterized as *caring* are mutually defined and can provide growth opportunities for both the student and the teacher. In fact, Gillespie (2002) proposed that such relationships can be transforming to the individual (both student and teacher) and even life affirming. *Reciprocal connecting,* characterized by authenticity and shared engagement, has a positive influence on learning outcomes in nursing (McGregor, 2005). This phrase implies that teachers and students know the other as human persons and respect and value each others' point of view. It eases the student–teacher interaction, allowing the student to better focus on learning without worrying about pleasing the teacher, focusing on clock hours and procedures (tasks), or knowing the right answer.

Connecting to students through relationship is accomplished in the classroom, online, and, most importantly, clinically. It is in this practice setting where a sense of caring professionalism is internalized, teamwork is learned, safety and quality are ensured, accountability is developed, and an appreciation for the larger system is formed. Clinical education is where the practice is showcased, and it offers faculty members the opportunity to role model, invite thinking, create safe space for exploration, and evaluate the effectiveness of their teaching.

Lately, however, clinical education is often relegated to part-timers and even staff nurses and is frequently looked down upon by tenure-track nursing faculty as a hindrance to more important research activities. There are few rewards and oftentimes disincentives for clinical education. Complicating this is the challenge of *teaching* caring. How does one teach a philosophical stance or, more aptly put, a way of being that is viewed by many as light, unscientific, or incongruent with present-day health care?

CARING PEDAGOGIES

Pedagogy refers to the art of teaching that encompasses specific methods, strategies, and instructional technologies.

> A caring pedagogy utilizes the caring factors (see chapter 2) to create an environment of engagement that is genuine and student-centered. *Caring,* as one of the core values of professional nursing, is honored, given high regard, and lived through the behaviors of faculty and staff. Faculty members who continuously reflect on the nature of nursing, themselves as teachers, and integrate the caring value of nursing with their words and actions set the tone of a school and become powerful role models for students.

According to Smith, Sheppard, Johnson, and Johnson (2005), who commented on the text *What Matters in College: Four Critical Years Revisited* (Astin, 1993), the interaction between faculty and students along with peer interaction "affected more general education outcomes than any other environmental variables . . . including the curriculum content" (pp. 1–2).

In this way of learning, covering all content areas during a program's short time frame is not possible. Rather, concepts central to the profession (such as caring) must be learned in depth and advanced over time with gradually increasing expectations of performance. Likewise, evaluation of learning should examine deep understanding versus superficial knowledge of core concepts. Thus, competency is developed. Using the traditional domains of learning (Bloom, 1956), caring cognitive, psychomotor, and affective knowledge is gained by learner-centered activities/experiences that facilitate depth, connection, and context. The faculty member's role is to design, facilitate, and evaluate the learning experiences in the context of relationship.

The caring factors provide the groundwork for student–teacher relationships (see Table 8.1).

Mutual problem solving assists students in understanding how to approach and think about clinical situations. Providing some information, reframing students' perceptions, brainstorming together, and using back-and-forth active discourse with appropriate feedback, faculty members

Table 8.1

POTENTIAL STUDENT CONSEQUENCES ASSOCIATED WITH FACULTY-CARING BEHAVIORS

CARING FACTOR	POTENTIAL CONSEQUENCES
Mutual problem solving	Whole systems (big picture) thinking; clinical reasoning; evidence-based decision-making
Attentive reassurance	Possibility; hope for the future
Human respect	Dignity; sense of worth
Encouraging manner	Confidence in abilities
Appreciation of unique meanings	Feel understood
Healing environment	Comfortable
Basic human needs	Security, self-esteem, self-caring
Affiliation needs	Connected; significant learning experiences

Feel "Cared For"

Student Satisfaction

Improved Learning Outcomes

Personal Growth

Caring Professional Practice

help shape students' comprehension of specific knowledge. The faculty member caringly uses the relationship as the basis for learning by engaging and encouraging student-led participation. In Tang et al.'s study (2005), the highest rated item explaining students' perceptions of effective clinical instructors was "solves problems with students" (p. 189). This factor was also reported by patients ($N = 557$), explaining the percentage of the variance in caring (Duffy, Hoskins, & Seifert, 2007).

Attentive reassurance requires availability on the part of the teacher along with a positive outlook on student performance. Availability of faculty is always an issue for students and faculty because demanding work lives and lifestyles often interfere. It is important for faculty members to take a look at how often and in what ways they allow students access to them. Office hours may not be enough, especially for online students who often do not come to campus. Multiple ways to ensure regular access to faculty are paramount; likewise, faculty members who make a point to initiate conversations (using various means) are considered important to students (Leners & Sitzman, 2006). Paying attention to students' progress requires faculty members to slow down enough to listen and notice their behaviors. In a phenomenological study of caring in nursing education, Coyle-Rogers and Cramer (2005) highlighted how educators "cared enough to recognize in the student a need for supportive assistance" (p. 164). Noticing behaviors in students and following up are important aspects of this caring factor. Failing students, in particular, need special time and an open and confident stance. McGregor's (2005) case study on a failing nursing student was enlightening. Keeping open a future of possibility was the central theme in the student's attempt to "recover" from uncaring practices of a few nursing faculty members. Occasionally students will fail; faculty members who offer students other hopeful futures (suggest alternative courses or careers) can help students find meaning and strength in the process.

Human respect, or honoring the inherent worth of individuals and accepting them unconditionally, is a fundamental caring factor that conveys that people matter. All individuals want to feel significant in some way, so when faculty members acknowledge students by name, use appropriate touch, and remember that students are members of families and larger communities that they value, students learn the importance of human dignity.

Using an *encouraging manner* refers to the demeanor of the faculty member. It consists of the congruence between verbal and nonverbal messages, showing enthusiasm for student activities, cheering for students, and providing appropriate positive feedback. This last behavior is frequently missed as faculty members assess examinations (particularly multiple-choice tests) and scholarly papers looking for mistakes or weaknesses in the student's work. Taking an alternative approach, choosing essay-type or other more reflective evaluation methods, and looking for the strengths and pointing out the good aspects of students' work take more time but promote confidence and build independence.

Appreciating the unique meanings or what is important to students is a caring factor that requires intention on the part of nursing faculty. This factor honors the individuality of each student and his/her background, culture, and life experiences. At the graduate level, using the varied nursing experiences of students in seminar discussions recognizes the expertise of students and enhances learning. Directing attention to students or staying student-centered is a purposeful behavior that is especially difficult when faculty members have large class sizes or online courses. Yet, recognizing the unique frame of reference of students, acknowledging their subjective perceptions, and using these to devise meaningful learning experiences avoid speculation and enhance further interactions.

Creating and maintaining a caring, healing environment in schools of nursing is a vital role for faculty administrators; but, individual faculty members are cocreators of that environment as they go about interacting with students, staff, and other faculty members. As the predominant setting where learning is taking place, maintaining surroundings that are conducive to learning is comforting to students and may reduce their anxiety. Such actions as maintaining a safe and confidential student lounge, providing adequate lighting, reducing noise, keeping safety a priority, resolving conflicts or disputes early, and bringing together experts or resources that augment classroom activities provide students with a caring milieu that enhances learning. The organizational culture or tone of the school, including the teamwork among faculty and staff, the vibrancy of employees, certain behavioral norms, and traditions, adds to the circumstances surrounding learning and has an impact on student performance. For example, faculty members in one school of nursing host a journal club once a month. By hosting this meeting, faculty demonstrate the importance of research by taking the time to coach a student leader who chooses and distributes an article and leads the discussion. The faculty member advises the student in the process and provides a safe space for dialogue. Another example is the discussions that faculty members and students have about patient situations in the clinical setting. A caring faculty member will consistently provide secure areas for students to respond to questions, inquire, and share ideas in confidence. Maintaining student confidentiality is important to future interactions and creates one of the conditions necessary for high-quality learning.

Meeting students' *basic human needs* is a caring factor that, on the face of it, doesn't seem pertinent to young, healthy persons. Yet, as individuals, physical, safety, social/relational, and self-esteem needs are important. It is critical that faculty members remember that basic human needs provide the motivation for behavior (Maslow, 1943). Adequate fluid and nutrition, rest and sleep, and exercise are physical needs that remain important during the educational process. Maintaining social relationships such as including students in group activities preserves belonging needs, while a sense of security provides order. In clinical situations, making sure students get to lunch, are working in a safe environment, and are recognized for their achievements meets basic human needs. Helping students learn to meet these needs through self-caring activities such as specific health promotion activities contributes to the students' future caring capacity. Keeping in mind that students have *affiliation needs* and belong to larger family and community groups is also caring in nature. When faculty members allow students to remain engaged in these groups through specific behaviors (e.g., allowing a student in a community-health course to complete a project for her own community), students may find more significance in their assignments and acquire more in-depth knowledge. Using the full range of caring factors provides quality learning experiences that may have profound consequences on student learning outcomes (see Table 8.1).

Within the framework of the Quality-Caring Model© (Duffy & Hoskins, 2003), innovative nurse educators are crafting learning objectives, courses, skills training, competencies, and values-based experiences using various instructional techniques to enhance nursing students' learning outcomes. For example, in the cognitive domain, objectives such as

1. Describe the multiple dimensions of relationship-centered caring including interdependence, community, and cultural competence;
2. Interpret the human experience of health and illness and its various meanings among diverse populations;
3. Identify the nature of caring relationships;
4. Examine the philosophical/theoretical foundations of relationship-centered caring;
5. Analyze the threats to the integrity of caring relationships, including social and cultural differences, and characteristics of the caregiver, the patient, and the health care system;
6. Synthesize information from caring theory, practice, and research findings in the relevant literature; and
7. Develop a plan for professional development including strategies to enhance self-awareness, the capacity for regular reflection, and continuous learning

were developed to provide a comprehensive course on relationship-centered caring (The Catholic University of America, 2006). Using multiple forms of experiential activities and evaluation techniques, students began to learn the meaning of professional caring. Classroom activities in this course were varied and experiential with active, participative learning. For example, caring factors were comprehended through a game of "Factor Feud," and small-group role playing was used to contrast caring and noncaring nursing practices. Multifaceted, problem-based case studies were used to develop plans of care applying the caring factors as intervention strategies. In addition, self-reflective exercises were assigned to augment classroom activities and promote integration of the concept.

Related to the psychomotor domain, students should be expected to perceive, recognize, and appropriately use caring behaviors (verbal and nonverbal) and to develop increasingly higher levels of caring professional practice. An appropriate objective for this domain might be: *practice human interaction skills, such as active listening, to initiate and cultivate caring relationships.* In one hospital using the Quality-Caring Model as their professional practice model, a required annual competency was developed to reinforce the quality of patient interactions (see Table 8.2). This competency included a case study followed by nursing actions that were videotaped so nurses could learn how to improve their caring practice. Another more impressive approach to this learning domain was reported by the Minnesota Baccalaureate Psychomotor Skills Faculty Group (2008). In this multisite study, investigators used the well-known blood pressure measurement as a way to integrate caring behaviors into a professional psychomotor skill. First, they revised the behaviors usually assessed during blood pressure skill evaluation to incorporate caring behaviors such as "faces client throughout procedure, maintains eye contact, voice is congruent with patient's emotions, physical contact is performed with a gentle touch" into the procedure (p. 102). To test the question, "is there a change in objective and subjective caring behaviors demonstrated by baccalaureate nursing students completing blood pressure measurement when those behaviors are taught in a nursing psychomotor skill curricula" (p. 101), they observed students before and after a demonstration of blood pressure measurement using caring behaviors, after completing an assigned reading, and after receiving caring content in the classroom using a variety of methods. Posttest scores ($N = 59$) were significantly higher ($F = 47.18$; $p < .000$) than pretest scores on objective caring behaviors. Increases in subjective scores were also present. These findings add to the notion of professional caring skill acquisition as developmental, that is, learned over time and in context. Faculty members were innovative in intentionally integrating caring professional practice within a common psychomotor skill. This intervention is very similar to the practice situation where nurses continuously blend psychomotor skills with cognitive and affective dimensions of practice (*being* and *doing* together). In this study, the process of human caring was operationalized in an integrated fashion where human caring and a specialized technique worked together to provide caring professional practice.

Table 8.2

COMPETENCY: PURPOSEFUL INTERACTION

PERFORMANCE CRITERIA	EVALUATION	RESOURCES & REMEDIATION	VALIDATOR INITIALS & DATE COMPLETED
Knocks on patient's door before entering the room	■ Case Scenario with demonstration or discussion	■ *See reference list	
Reviews white board with patient's information	■ Observation in daily work experience		
Sits down next to patient	■ Role Play		
Maintains eye contact	■ Discussion		
Touches the patient lightly on the hand— if appropriate			
Sits leaning slightly forward facing the patient			
Ensures choice of words, tone, and body language all convey the same meaning			
Listens intently to the patient			

(Continued)

Table 8.2

COMPETENCY: PURPOSEFUL INTERACTION (*Continued*)

PERFORMANCE CRITERIA	EVALUATION	RESOURCES & REMEDIATION	VALIDATOR INITIALS & DATE COMPLETED
Acknowledges the patient with subtle changes in expressions and/or nodding the head			
Uses active listening techniques— repeating, reflection, and empathy			
Speaks to patient in a calm, respectful, and clear voice			
Uses open-ended questions			
Responds to the feeling tone of the patient			
Encourages sharing of feelings			
Suggests coping strategies if appropriate			
Brings closure to the conversation and follows through on any issues			
Documents the purposeful interaction			

In the affective domain of learning, students are expected to value, appropriately respond, and eventually internalize important professional concepts. Values-based experiential activities such as service learning or participating in caring groups help students accept and embrace the importance of caring as the cornerstone for professional nursing practice. One school of nursing approached this aspect of learning by incorporating a model of affective development that guided the process of internalizing the concept *caring* over the course of the entire curriculum (Cook & Cullen, 2003). By setting a caring nursing educational environment, carefully planned and selected teaching/learning strategies, and multiple assessment approaches, the faculty successfully assisted Associate Degree students to internalize caring as the dominant theme in professional nursing practice.

Another approach to helping nursing students internalize the significance of their emerging nursing practice is to help them think about or interpret their relationships with patients and families. According to their hermeneutical study, Ironside and Diekelmann (2005) found that students referred to times when they were able to make a difference as "knowing and connecting." Engaged groups of students and teachers jointly unraveling descriptions of their experiences help both students and teachers discover important factors about what and how students are learning nursing practice.

Online education and new graduate orientation are two areas where caring relationships between students and faculty are not usually mentioned. However, the question of how to effectively convey caring in these student populations is a significant one. In two qualitative reports, a team of researchers explored the question of student perceptions of caring in online baccalaureate and graduate education (Leners & Sitzman, 2006; Sitzman & Leners, 2006). Similar themes of empathy, frequent feedback, timeliness, tone of appreciation, and being committed or able to "feel the passion of caring online" emerged from the data (Leners & Sitzman, 2006, p. 315). Particularly from the graduate students' perspectives, faculty members' choice of words and punctuation had great significance for student morale. It conveyed the encouragement needed to continue in the course. In general, frequency, availability, and immediacy of interaction were attributed to caring as was the students' need for faculty to know them personally. Primarily in baccalaureate students, faculty caring was necessary to convey that the online students were just as important as the classroom students. Although limited by the methods and samples, these studies contribute to the idea that intentional caring in online education can enhance learning.

Continuing to perfect caring professional practice after graduation is a lifelong effort, but the new graduate experience can contribute or thwart such practice. In a phenomenological study of caring behaviors of preceptors (Schumacher, 2007), data were collected from journal entries and in-depth interviews. Findings included six caring and four noncaring themes between preceptors and new graduate orientees. Advocating, welcoming, including, preceptor presence, genuine feedback, and human-to-human connections were described as caring interactions by orientees. Such behaviors as taking time to make sure assignments were good learning experiences, asking questions, listening, using an open and approachable demeanor, including orientees in unit activities and committees, being physically present without hovering, and sharing some of the deeper rules of the professional nursing culture were listed as caring. Unfortunately, the noncaring interactions were described as unwelcoming (no eye contact, no introduction to the unit), underpresence of preceptor (did not check on orientees, allowing them to make serious patient errors), overpresence of preceptor such that they did everything for the orientee, and noncaring feedback (unclear, confusing, conflicting, or not authentic). These experiences have important implications for staff development educators, preceptors, and nursing leaders. Caring relationships between preceptors and orientees are necessary to make successful transitions between the educational role and professional practice and are linked to retention of new nurses (Nursing Executive Center, 2002). Preceptors should be chosen and educated carefully and model caring behaviors, helping new nursing graduates better implement caring professional practice.

ASSURING CARING COMPETENCY

Competency is a complex phenomenon referring to an individual's expertise and ability to perform a skillset in a particular discipline. Competency in nursing has been defined as the formal exhibition of a skill, ability, or aptitude of a professional nurse (Meretoja & Leino-Kilpi, 2001). As such, its measurement is daunting and requires multiple approaches. It is best accomplished by assessing an individual's ability to demonstrate identified behaviors (competency statements or competencies) in the practice setting. Competency statements in nursing typically relate to the three learning domains and are scored based on some pre-established criteria (Bloom, 1956).

Competency assessment has undergone significant debate in nursing education over the years because it conflicts with a basic premise of higher education, that is, lifelong learning. University faculty believe their goal is to prepare beginning practitioners who are lifelong learners, while employers want graduates who can immediately perform upon employment, who are aware of workplace needs, and who have more than beginning competence. Thus, ensuring competency is seen as limiting by some faculty and yet necessary by nursing leaders as they try to uphold an environment of quality and safety in clinical agencies. So, despite the fact that graduates of nursing programs are expected to initiate, cultivate, and sustain caring relationships with their patients and members of the health care team (Duffy & Hoskins, 2003), caring competency in nursing is rarely measured summatively in the academic setting and even less so in the practice environment (Duffy, 2005; Sadler, 2003). Starting with a definition of caring and a competency framework that includes all components of registered nurse performance, however, statements demonstrating caring knowledge, abilities, and values can be identified and used for evaluative purposes. Statements reflecting generic knowledge of caring relationships might include the following.

The new graduate/beginning registered nurse:

Demonstrates an understanding of the relationship of caring to quality health care

Recognizes that caring relationships are driven by the needs of patients and their families

Contributes to the practice environment to maximize relationship-centered caring

Uses caring factors in the delivery of patient care

Recognizes that feeling "cared for" is "what matters" to patients and families

Values caring as the primary role of the nurse

An example of more specific competencies for beginning staff nurses can be found in Table 8.3.

Table 8.3

BEGINNING STAFF-NURSE CARING COMPETENCIES FOR PROFESSIONAL PRACTICE

ASSESSMENT	Initiates a caring relationship with patient/family
	Performs comprehensive assessments on patients/families using a holistic framework
	Conducts routine patient checks throughout patient's length of stay
	Integrates multiple "ways of knowing" to gather pertinent patient information
	Identification
	Mutually identifies measurable outcomes for patients/families
	Identifies possible psychosocio/cultural/spiritual and legal/ethical/fiscal issues that may interfere with caring relationships
	Identifies priorities of care
PLAN	In partnership with the patient and family, develops a comprehensive plan of care
	In partnership with the patient and family, revises the plan as indicated
	Recognizes patient/family rights and preferences in the development of plan of care
	Designs holistic nursing interventions
	Plans for continuity and discharge needs
IMPLEMENT	Accurately performs nursing interventions using the following caring factors:
	Human Respect
	Recognizes and accepts patients' inherent dignity
	Treats patients and families kindly
	Actively listens to patient and family concerns
	Demonstrates unconditional human respect
	Attentive Reassurance
	Remains available to patients and families
	Expresses interest in patients and families

(Continued)

Table 8.3

BEGINNING STAFF-NURSE CARING COMPETENCIES FOR PROFESSIONAL PRACTICE (*Continued*)

Reinforces patients'/families' sense of hope

Anticipates patients' needs and preferences

Encouraging Manner

Supports patients and families in their beliefs

Offers realistic optimism

Encourages patients and families to ask questions

Assists patients to deal with bad feelings

Allows patients and families to make decisions

Encourages patients/families to continue with their health care

Healing Environment

Routinely checks up on patients/families

Pays attention to patients/families

Assists patients to feel as comfortable as possible

Respects patient and family privacy

Creates safe, orderly, predictable, and aesthetically pleasing surroundings

Treats the physical body carefully

Mutual Problem Solving

Assists patients and families to understand their own thinking

Questions patients and families about their treatment

Assists patients and families with alternate ways of dealing with their illness/es

Assesses patients' and families' knowledge

Assists patients/families to figure out questions to ask their health care providers

Appreciation of Unique Meanings

Demonstrates concern about how patients/families view their health care

Discerns what is important to patients and families

(Continued)

Table 8.3

**BEGINNING STAFF-NURSE CARING COMPETENCIES
FOR PROFESSIONAL PRACTICE (*Continued*)**

	Acknowledges patients' feelings
	Shows regard for what has meaning to patients and families
	Basic Human Needs
	Ensures patients' physical needs are met, including food and fluids, elimination, sleep and rest, mobility, hygiene, ventilation, sensory stimulation, and solitude
	Assists patients and families to feel less worried
	Upholds patients' sense of independence
	Affiliation Needs
	Ensures contact with significant others is preserved
	Responsive to patients' family
	Communicates with patients' family
	Involves family in health care decisions as desired by the patient
EVALUATE	Demonstrates an awareness of patient outcomes
	Utilizes a creative problem-solving approach to address ongoing patient problems
	Routinely assesses patients' responses to care and achievement of outcomes; revises plan of care accordingly

Other aspects of the professional nursing role might be considered by the following competency statements:

Professional Relationships

Collaborates with other health care providers in designing and providing care to patients and their families

Communicates using the caring factors to create a positive working environment

Tailors verbal and written communication based on sociocultural, spiritual, knowledge, literacy, and preferred language

Using the caring factors, facilitates problem solving among the health care team

Using the caring factors, effectively delegates and supervises assistive personnel

Supports the holistic development of colleagues

Assumes a leadership role in meeting patient and family needs

Creates a sense of teamwork—offers assistance to coworkers

Uses relevant leadership/management strategies to guide improvements in the health care system

Provides useful feedback to health care team members in a caring manner

Establishes and maintains caring relationships among the health care team beyond the department

Acknowledges others' strengths

Willingly offers assistance to other staff who are stressed or need breaks from the work environment

Professional Decision Making

Concurrently, uses best available evidence to make sound clinical judgments

Maintains awareness of one's own biases that may influence judgments

Uses all sources of knowledge (research, standards, experience, etc.) as evidence for clinical decision-making

Maintains technological competence in order to access best available evidence

Independently, continuously updates knowledge using current research

Professionalism

Practices in accordance with established ethical and legal standards

Advocates for patients and their families' needs, rights, and preferences

Sets standards of human caring

Interprets and responds to ethical issues in the workplace using appropriate channels

Contributes to the improvement of the internal and external health care system through research

Demonstrates self-awareness through ongoing reflection and critical examination

Uses this information for self-caring

Uses centering practices through the work shift to refocus energies on patients and families

Role models and advocates healthy behaviors

Ensures accurate, comprehensive, and timely communication

Uses appropriate written communication

Remains open to feedback in order to advance learning and professional growth

Uses health care resources wisely

Demonstrates accountability for responsibilities delegated to assistive personnel

Seeks ways to participate in institution-wide activities such as shared leadership, quality improvement, and other committees

Examines competency of practice annually, identifying strengths as well as areas of professional development

Develops annual goals and action plans for achieving them

Maintains and holds oneself and others accountable for human caring practices

While competencies can be useful, their measurement is complicated and does not guarantee continued expert performance. One organization using a caring professional practice model developed caring competencies in the traditional Benner (1984) novice-to-expert approach and uses the more advanced behaviors in their professional development program (clinical ladder) to advance professional nurses at the bedside.

In this approach, the novice nurse is considered more task-oriented and has beginning understanding of caring relationships. The advanced beginner interacts with patients and families using caring behaviors, but in-depth use is not evident. The competent nurse connects with complex patients and colleagues in a caring manner, is beginning to recognize and act on self-caring needs, and ensures a human caring environment. The proficient nurse knows his/her patients and families and can anticipate their needs. He/she cultivates caring relationships among the health care team and role models caring. The expert nurse is fully grounded in caring and has advanced skills in caring relationships. He/she is able to care for self as well as patients and families, contributes through caring relationships to the local and professional communities, and serves as a caring leader in the department and the organization.

While these examples provide models for caring competency identification, they are limited because their evaluation is completed in only one perspective, that of the supervisor. A comprehensive approach using the 360-degree method (Edwards & Ewen, 1996; London & Smither, 1995), where caring competency is assessed from the perspective of the one being evaluated (nurse self-evaluation), those being "cared for" (patients and families), the supervisor, and colleagues (other nurses, physicians, other members of the health care team), provides a more thorough evaluation of nurse caring capacity. By its very nature, 360-degree evaluation is relationship-centered, using the wisdom of multiple sources and perspectives to provide important feedback. Using this approach, self-evaluation of caring can be accomplished quantitatively with established valid and reliable tools (Caring Ability Inventory [CAI], Nkongho, 1990; Caring Efficacy Scale [CES], Coates, 1997) and/or qualitatively through reflective analysis. Within a school of nursing, Sadler (2003) used the Caring Efficacy Scale to measure self-reported caring competency of baccalaureate students in seven classes representing differing program levels and found no differences in caring competency among the groups. Furthermore, final semester seniors reported the role modeling of their parents as contributing most to their development of caring capacity. Unfortunately, out of 28 graduating seniors, only 4 students specifically wrote about the contribution of the nursing curriculum as a factor in their caring capacity.

Evaluation of caring capacity from the patient's perspective offers unique insights into how patients view professional nursing practice and can assist nurses to better understand how to improve their practice. Determining how patients and their families perceive students' interactions is a direct measure of their (students') ability to translate the concept of caring to the bedside. Applying this approach, Duffy (2005) used the Caring Assessment Tool (CAT) with senior baccalaureate students as one method to evaluate their caring competency. In this study, students were expected (under the supervision of their clinical instructor) to obtain feedback using the CAT from three patients during their final clinical course. Patient narratives were invited by a one-item question added to the tool to provide a rich in-depth approach to this assessment. Findings demonstrated that patients viewed the students as having above-average caring capacity overall, but three distinct areas, namely spiritual support, responding honesty, and helping patients understand their sexuality, were rated lower.

Competency evaluation using the 360-degree method, while more holistic, is complicated because once competency statements are identified, a measurement rubric must be developed and then determined to be psychometrically sound, data gathered (using appropriate sampling methods) and analyzed, and feedback offered to the student/employee. The application of this method is cumbersome for both staff or student and administrators or faculty members; however, some evidence from the management literature does suggest that 360-degree feedback is helpful in setting improvement goals and advancing performance (Edwards & Ewen, 1996). In nursing, one might use the feedback from such a comprehensive evaluation in both academia and the clinical setting to encourage more open dialogue about caring professional practice, reinforce the importance of caring behaviors, reflect back to the recipient how significant their practice is to patient outcomes, identify strengths and areas for development, and raise awareness of faculty and nurse leaders of how the curriculum or the environment might be influencing caring practice. Much more research is needed to determine if this approach will improve nursing students' and practicing nurses' caring capacity.

PROGRAM EVALUATION: IMPLEMENTING THE QUALITY-CARING MODEL FOR EDUCATION

Summative evaluation of concepts considered central to a program's curriculum and based on that program's philosophy and objectives provides important evidence of programmatic success. Such evaluation helps meet the mandate of producing competent clinicians who can fulfill practice expectations. One such practice expectation is caring. In a caring educational environment using a caring-based curriculum, it would follow that a quality program evaluation would encompass caring learning outcomes. A framework for program evaluation helps guide the assessment process. To that end, an adaptation of the Quality-Caring Model was proposed (Figure 8.1). The Quality-Caring Model for Educational Program Evaluation is dynamic and evidence-based (Duffy, 2005). The model helps to identify structure and process variables that contribute to educational outcomes. In this model, the *structure* component includes characteristics of faculty, students, and the educational system. Concepts and subconcepts included in this component may directly or indirectly influence educational outcomes. The *process* component includes

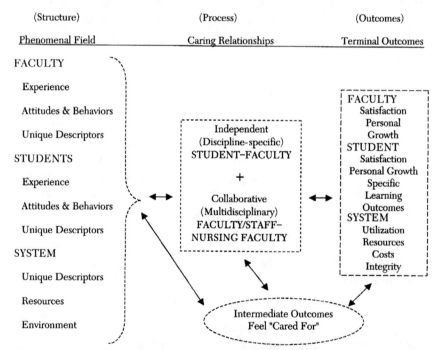

Figure 8.1 Quality-Caring Model for Educational Program Evaluation©. Adapted from the Quality-Caring Model© (Duffy & Hoskins, 2003).

From "Want to Graduate Nurses Who Care?" by J. Duffy, 2005, in M. H. Oermann & K. T. Heinrich (Eds.), *Annual Review of Nursing Educational Research, 3,* 59–76.

the two essential caring relationships that comprise the work of nursing faculty. The independent relationship between students and faculty is primary and includes values, attitudes, and behaviors that faculty members carry out in partnership with students during the learning process. Such relationships undergird and facilitate student learning, leading to specific educational outcomes.

Collaborative relationships include those activities and responsibilities that nursing faculty members share with other faculty members and administrative personnel throughout a university system. Meetings, task forces, and coordinating activities among university departments represent many disciplines working together in collaborative relationships that ultimately lead to shared educational outcomes. For example, a nursing department and the theater department may work together to develop and teach a course for nursing students where student actors are also involved. Such planning is collaborative and enriches quality educational outcomes.

The third major component of the model, *outcomes,* corresponds to the end result of the educational process. Two forms of outcomes are apparent. Intermediate outcomes represent a change in behaviors, emotions, or knowledge, while terminal outcomes are those major end-result concepts that affect the future of a program. Intermediate outcomes often include attainment of specific course learning goals but also can include feelings about the learning process. Of importance is the intermediate outcome—feeling cared for. "When one feels 'cared for,' a sense of security develops making it easier to learn, change behaviors, and take risks" (Duffy & Hoskins, 2003, p. 83). Students who feel cared for while in the learning environment have reported less anxiety and more skill acquisition (Pullen et al., 2001). Although not reported in the literature, faculty who feel cared for in the work environment may report increased job satisfaction.

The major proposition of the model is that relationships characterized by caring contribute to positive educational outcomes. Furthermore, the structure-process-outcomes components are a function of time and circumstance and are dynamic. Ongoing feedback and revisions are consistent with a continuous search for excellence.

With a foundational model as a guide, a program's evaluation plan should reflect the faculty's decisions about responsibility, frequency of assessment, specific measurements, and acceptable criteria. Multiple perspectives applied formatively over the course of the curriculum, culminating in end-of-program summative evaluation, are recommended.

Measuring nurse caring can be accomplished from the perspective of the student, the faculty, and, most importantly, the recipients of caring (patients).

Although subjective, student self-reports of nurse caring can provide a baseline assessment at program entry and then be followed annually (or more frequently) to determine improvement. This allows for trending by program level and over time. Choosing instruments that are practical and have established psychometric properties is essential. From the students' perspective, self-assessment data can be gathered on admission and then annually thereafter to compare growth.

Clinical evaluation tools that include an objective measure of nurse caring that is consistent across the program can be used from a faculty perspective to assess students' progress in caring competence. Such a measure can be as simple as one item with higher scores expected as students progress in the program or composed of multiple items that are summed for a total score. Faculty evaluation of students' caring competencies can then be easily assessed in each clinical course and compared across the program.

Patients' perceptions of student nurse-caring capacity are important to better evaluate whether students are actually conveying caring to patients and families. To prevent faculty and patient burden, a limited number of these evaluations is recommended at key points in a program. Using valid and reliable instruments, faculty can design how students will best select patients and administer the instrument. Scores from such evaluations should be shared with students and used by faculty (along with the other evaluations) to provide feedback about performance and make judgments about the effectiveness of the curriculum in preparing caring graduates.

Students' perceptions of faculty-caring behaviors (e.g., feeling "cared for") can be assessed using established instruments. As noted in the literature review, creating caring environments during the educational process and role-modeling caring seem to raise awareness and facilitate learning. Assessing students' perceptions of faculty caring can yield important data about the structure and processes of the educational program. The Caring Assessment Tool–Educational Version (CAT-edu) is an example instrument used for evaluating this valuable educational outcome (Duffy, 2003). Students can complete this at the end of their program, and results can be used to revise faculty members' interactions with future students.

While this discussion has centered on quantitative program evaluation, using qualitative approaches such as reflective journaling, narratives, portfolios, focus groups, and other methods adds valuable information to the quantitative assessment. Lastly, correlating structure and process variables such as student demographics or faculty credentials with specific learning outcomes provides data that can be used to adjust learning outcomes and for policy revision.

SUMMARY

This chapter focused on teaching and learning the practice of nursing. In particular, student–teacher relationships are highlighted. Through role modeling and using caring pedagogies that are student-centered, faculty members can design meaningful learning experiences that contribute to positive learning outcomes. The relationship between teacher and student can be growth-producing for both and encompasses classroom, online, and clinical settings. The caring factors provide the framework for student–teacher caring relationships, encouraging openness, risk-taking, and engagement. Incorporating aspects of these factors into specific learning objectives best integrates the concept of caring as the key ingredient in professional practice. Caring competencies when developed and assessed in a comprehensive manner can be useful in helping students and practicing nurses become more aware of the importance of caring professional practice. Finally, using the Quality-Caring Model for Education as a guide, schools of nursing can incorporate caring assessments formatively and summatively to ensure that this important value is embedded in both the curriculum and the environment and students' progress is followed.

CALLS TO ACTION

Student–faculty caring relationships combined with faculty role modeling during the educational process are the best possible

(continued)

ways to help students learn professional caring. **Evaluate** your relationships with students.

Using the context of caring relationships to design and implement learning experiences assists nursing students to understand complex phenomena. Faculty members who connect caring nursing situations to the larger whole enable graduates to adjust to the complex health care system and transfer their knowledge to a variety of nursing situations. **Increase** the amount of time you spend with students this week.

The performance of nursing is best demonstrated during clinical education. In the clinical situation, faculty members have the opportunity to encourage opinions, shape ideas, establish a secure system for inquiry, and assess the usefulness of their teaching. **Sign up** for a clinical course.

Noticing students' attitudes and actions, actively listening to verbal and behavioral cues, and showing interest in their work are necessary to gauge student progress. It requires faculty members to remain unhurried, focused, and deliberate enough to pay attention. **Acknowledge** the strengths of students' work.

Professional nurses are better able to advance their practice (and resulting caring capacity) when they receive information from the patient's perspective. Such detail offers unique insight directly from the source and suggests specific ways to improve. **Rewrite** your last lecture to include the patient's perspective.

In the context of caring relationships, nursing faculty members have the responsibility to design, facilitate, and evaluate learning experiences that positively impact student learning and enhance patient outcomes. **Revise** your student evaluation method/s to enhance student learning.

Important information about an educational organization and its curriculum can be obtained by assessing students' perceptions of faculty caring. **Use** a valid and reliable tool to measure students' perceptions of faculty caring upon graduation.

Reflective Questions/Applications for Students

1. Discuss what it means to be a practice discipline.
2. How did you learn "to care"? How do you keep this knowledge current?
3. What reflective learning activities are you engaged in? How would you evaluate and/or revise them?
4. Define integrative learning.
5. Describe the components of caring pedagogies.
6. Analyze the term *competency* as it relates to caring capacity.

Reflective Questions/Applications for Educators

7. Review Schon's (1987) work on understanding a practice discipline. How can you adapt some of its important principles in your work?
8. Appraise the phrase *integrative learning*. How is it operationalized in your curriculum?
9. Evaluate whether caring pedagogies are fully applied in your institution. What could you do to better implement them?
10. List baccalaureate and graduate student demands that limit authentic relationships in the educational environment. How could these be eased or the environment revised to enhance relationship building?
11. What caring and noncaring faculty behaviors do you observe at your institution?
12. Analyze the core concepts that undergird your curriculum. How are they learned in depth and advanced over the program? What evaluation methods do you use to ensure profound understanding of these concepts?
13. What innovative strategies can you identify to ensure the three domains of learning related to caring are threaded throughout your curriculum?
14. How would you implement a 360-degree student evaluation program in your curriculum?
15. Reflect on your role as a faculty member. How do you role-model caring? What self-caring practices do you regularly carry out? Are you certain that meaningful (i.e., breadth and depth of the content) learning occurs in your classroom? What ways can you identify to integrate caring pedagogies into your teaching style?

16. Make a list of the caring factors and describe how you enact them in relationships with baccalaureate and graduate students. Do they differ based on level? Should they?

17. Consider an online course with graduate students. Develop at least three learning objectives each for the cognitive, psychomotor, and affective domains that include caring relationships. How would you ensure by your interactions with students that caring was conveyed?

18. Consider a course that you currently teach. As a student-centered course with small groups of engaged learners, design a caring learning experience that includes five small (3–5 students) groups each with its own activity that blends into one larger caring concept.

19. What ideas do you have to help baccalaureate students develop deep meanings of the caring relationships they have with patients and families? How would you implement them? What practice experiences could best provide opportunities for students to know and connect with patients and families?

20. What strategies might you use with graduate students to help them develop deep meanings regarding the caring relationships they should cultivate with the health care team? How would you implement them?

21. What type of faculty members can best utilize caring pedagogies? Are there some who can't? What are the characteristics of those who are successful?

22. Describe how you are able to transfer humanness from the simulation lab to the clinical area.

Reflective Questions/Applications for Nurse Leaders

23. How does the new graduate experience at your institution affect caring professional practice?

24. What continuing education activities at your institution promote caring professional practice?

25. Are nurse-caring behaviors integrated into the required annual competencies at your institution? Could they be integrated? How would you go about revising them?

REFERENCES

American Nurses Association. (2003). *The social policy statement for nurses.* Washington, DC: Author.

Astin, A. (1993). *What matters in college? Four critical years revisited.* San Francisco, CA: Jossey-Bass.

Beck, C. T. (2001). Caring within nursing education: A metasynthesis. *Journal of Nursing Education, 40,* 101–109.

Benner, P. (1984). *From novice to expert: Excellence and power in clinical nursing practice* (Commemorative ed.). Old Tappan, NJ: Addison Wesley Publishing Company.

Bevis, E. O., & Watson, J. (1989). *Toward a caring curriculum: A new pedagogy for nursing.* New York: National League for Nursing Press.

Bloom, B. S. (1956). *Taxonomy of educational objectives, Handbook I: The cognitive domain.* New York: David McKay Co. Inc.

The Catholic University of America. (2006). *Nursing 567: Relationship-centered caring.* Washington, DC: Author.

Coates, C. J. (1997). The caring efficacy scale: Nurses self-reports of caring in practice settings. *Advanced Practice Nursing Quarterly, 3*(1), 53–59.

Cook, P. R., & Cullen, J. A. (2003). Caring as an imperative for nursing education. *Nursing Education Perspectives, 24*(4), 192–197.

Coyle-Rogers, P., & Cramer, M. (2005). The phenomenon of caring: The perspectives of nurse educators. *Journal for Nurses in Staff Development, 21*(4), 160–170.

Duffy, J. (2003). Caring assessment tools. In J. Watson (Ed.), *Instruments for assessing and measuring caring in nursing and health sciences.* New York: Springer Publishing.

Duffy, J. (2005). Want to graduate nurses who care?: Assessing nursing students' caring competencies. *Annual Review of Nursing Education, 3,* 73–97.

Duffy, J., & Hoskins, L. (2003). The Quality-Caring Model©: Blending dual paradigms. *Advances in Nursing Science, 26*(1), 77–88.

Duffy, J., Hoskins, L. M., & Seifert, R. F. (2007). Dimensions of caring: Psychometric properties of the Caring Assessment Tool. *Advances in Nursing Science, 30*(3), 235–245.

Edgerton, R. (2001). *Education white paper.* Pew Forum on Undergraduate Learning. Retrieved May 2, 2008, from http://www.pewundergradforum.org/wp1html

Edwards, M., & Ewen, A. J. (1996). *360 degree feedback: The powerful new model for employee assessment & performance improvement.* New York: American Management Association.

Fawcett, J. (1984). *Analysis and evaluation of conceptual models of nursing.* Philadelphia, PA: FA Davis.

Gillespie, M. (2002). Student-teacher connection in clinical nursing education. *Journal of Advanced Nursing, 37,* 566–576.

Gramling, L., & Nugent, K. (1998). Teaching caring within the context of health. *Nurse Educator, 23*(2), 47–51.

Huber, M. T., Hutchings, P., Gale, R., Breen, M., & Miller, R. (2007). Leading initiatives for integrative learning. *Liberal Education, 93*(2), 57–60.

Inui, T. (2003). *A flag in the wind: Educating for professionalism in medicine.* Washington, DC: Association of American Medical Colleges.

Ironside, P., & Diekelmann, N. (2005). Learning the practices of knowing and connecting: The voices of students. *Journal of Nursing Education, 44*(4), 153–155.

Leach, D. C. (2002). Competence is a habit. *Journal of the American Medical Association, 287,* 243–244.

Leners, D. S., & Sitzman, K. (2006). Graduate student perceptions: Feeling the passion of CARING online. *Nursing Education Perspectives, 27*(6), 315–319.

London, M., & Smither, J. W. (1995). Can multisource feedback change perceptions of goal accomplishments, self-evaluations, and performance-related outcomes? Theory-based applications and directions for research. *Personnel Psychology, 48,* 803–839.

Maslow, A. H. (1943). A theory of human motivation. *Psychological Review, 50,* 370–396.

McGregor, A. (2005). Enacting connectedness in nursing education: Moving from pickets of rhetoric to reality. *Nursing Education Perspectives, 26*(2), 90–95.

Meretoja, R., & Leino-Kilpi, H. (2001). Instruments for evaluating nurse competence. *Journal of Nursing Administration, 31*(7/8), 346–352.

Minnesota Baccalaureate Psychomotor Skills Faculty Group. (2008). Nursing student caring behaviors during blood pressure measurement. *Journal of Nursing Education, 47*(3), 98–104.

Nkongho, N. (1990). The caring ability inventory. In O. Strickland & C. Waltz (Eds.), *Measurement of nursing outcomes.* New York: Springer Publishing.

Nursing Executive Center. (2002). *Destination nursing: Creating a destination hospital for nurses.* Washington, DC: The Advisory Board Company.

Poormann, S., Webb, C., & Mastorovich, M. L. (2002). Students' stories: How faculty help or hinder students at risk. *Nurse Educator, 27*(3), 126–131.

Pullen, R., Murray, P., & McGee, K. (2001). Care groups: A model to mentor novice nursing students/orientees. *Nurse Educator, 26*(6), 283–288.

Sadler, J. (2003). A pilot study to measure the caring efficacy of baccalaureate nursing students. *Nursing Education Perspectives, 24*(6), 295–299.

Schon, D. (1987). *Educating the reflective practitioner.* San Francisco: Jossey-Bass.

Schumacher, D. L. (2007). Caring behaviors of preceptors as perceived by new nursing graduate orientees. *Journal for Nurses in Staff Development, 23*(4), 186–192.

Sitzman, K., & Leners, D. W. (2006). Student perceptions of caring in online baccalaureate education. *Nursing Education Perspectives, 27*(9), 254–259.

Smith, K. A., Sheppard, S. D., Johnson, D. W., & Johnson, R. T. (2005, January). Pedagogies of engagement: Classroom-based practices. *Journal of Engineering Education,* 1–15.

Tang, F., Chou, S., & Chiang, H. (2005). Students' perceptions of effective and ineffective clinical instructors. *Journal of Nursing Education, 44*(4), 187–192.

Tanner, C. (1990). Reflections on the curriculum revolution. *Journal of Nursing Education, 29,* 295–299.

Watson, J. (1979). *Nursing: The philosophy and science of caring.* Denver: University of Colorado Press.

Wheatley, M. (2005). *Finding our way.* San Francisco: Berrett-Koehler Publishers.

Yordy, K. (2006). *The nursing faculty shortage: A crisis for health care.* Robert Wood Johnson Foundation. Retrieved May 2, 2008, from http://www.ahcnet.org/pdf/fac tors_affecting_the_health_workforce_2005.pdf

9

Evaluating and Researching Quality Caring

Somewhere, something incredible is waiting to be known.

—Dr. Carl Sagan

Keywords: measurement, caring, evaluation, caring science

MEASURING CARING

As a concept so central to professional nursing practice, demonstrating the value of caring is crucial, not only to the profession but to patients and their families and policymakers. While qualitative investigations have provided the meanings and patterns of caring as well as some caring theories, often quantitative data is needed to assess practice, evaluate programs or services, improve practice (quality improvement), provide evidence for decision-making, generate connections among variables, test caring interventions, and validate and refine theory. *Measurement*, a fundamental aspect of quantitative analysis, is generally understood as a process by which attributes or dimensions of a phenomenon are assigned a value (to eliminate guessing or uncertainty). Caring is measured when we want to identify its presence, determine how frequently it is occurring, how well it occurs, how important it is, what it is associated with, how it compares among groups, and persons' opinions of it. Using a systematic method of collecting data (to ensure accurate and consistent application) and employing focused instruments are implicit in measurement. Yet, measuring nursing phenomena is usually associated with some error—either in the instrument itself, how the data were collected, or in the characteristics of the sample. Reducing this error is a major goal of high-quality instruments.

Understanding how an instrument was developed is important because it has implications for its accuracy, application in practice, and interpretation of results. First, recognizing the definition or conceptual framework from which the items were generated is paramount. Multiple frameworks for understanding caring have been proposed (Boykin & Schoenhofer, 1993; Leininger, 1981; Roach, 1984; Swanson, 1991; Watson, 1979, 1985); therefore, appreciating the basic meaning of caring, which drove the item development, will help to clarify how findings can be interpreted. Second, the context in which the instrument was developed is crucial to understand. For example, the patient population, setting, age group of respondents, emotional states of respondents, and severity of illness all have a bearing on the results. Third, most instruments are created for a specific purpose, and using them for a different objective is problematic for interpretation. For example, a caring instrument designed to measure the *importance* of various caring behaviors would not be appropriate if the objective was to measure *how often* caring was occurring in a situation. In fact, the results would be suspect. Fourth, the perspective from which a phenomenon is being measured impacts results. For example, if one were measuring caring using a tool developed in an acute care setting, administering the same instrument to nurses who work in a school-based clinic may not necessarily yield the same results. Fifth, clarity of items, including the degree of readability, is important. If an item was meant to measure mutual problem solving, for example (a caring factor), but the way it was worded connoted trust, the answers would not necessarily be valid. Additionally, if items on a caring instrument were worded in language that was difficult to understand, respondents may not accurately be able to answer it. Finally, how an instrument is administered impacts its results—for example, potential biases of the data collector/s, burden to the patient (i.e., how long it took), consistency of administration, and interrater reliability (multiple data collectors using the same approach) all affect how an instrument performs. Obviously, validity (accuracy) and reliability (consistency) of instruments are a major concern, and these properties should be explicitly made known to potential users. (See Table 9.1 for a list of criteria from which to judge caring instruments.)

Table 9.1

CRITERIA FOR CHOOSING CARING INSTRUMENTS

CRITERIA	QUESTIONS FOR CONSIDERATION
Conceptual framework	On whose theory or conceptual base were the items developed?
Purpose	What was the original purpose of the instrument?
Context	In what patient population or setting has the instrument been used?
Perspective	From whose viewpoint is the tool seeking information—patients, families, students, or nurses?
Clarity	Are the items understandable? Are the directions easy?
Administration	What is the time required for completion? How is scoring accomplished?
Psychometrics	Is the tool valid and reliable? What forms of validity and reliability have been measured? Are they consistent with your purpose?

For further information on measurement and instrument development, see Nancy Burns and Susan K. Grove's *The Practice of Nursing Research: Conduct, Critique, and Utilization* (2005). The chapters on measurement and data collection (pp. 389–469) provide a good overview of quantifying variables, including reducing measurement error and ensuring accurate, reliable, and sensitive assessment. In the context of this brief background regarding measurement and instrument development pertaining to caring, the importance of choosing appropriate caring instruments with the most credibility is stressed. Because the phenomenon of caring has been conceptualized, it *is* measurable, and several tools already exist to aid in this process.

While many have attempted to measure caring (Watson, 2002), there remains confusion about how and what to measure. Beck (1999) completed a review of 11 caring instruments; they varied in terms of their scoring structure, conceptual definition of caring, the perspective from which it was answered (patients, nurses, or others), and psychometric properties. Furthermore, use of the instruments in various studies was limited by sample type and size. Beck recommended additional evaluation with rigorous sampling and psychometric analysis. Of the more than 21 instruments that measure caring in *Assessing and Measuring Caring in Nursing and Health Sciences* (Watson, 2002), only 7 measured caring from the patients' point of view. Different conceptualizations of caring were used, few focused on direct interpersonal behaviors linked to caring, and methods for testing reliability and validity were not explicit in some instruments. In a review of this text, Baumann (2003) suggested that while there are limitations in the use of quantitative measures to assess caring, the instruments as a whole do advance nursing.

Three recent instruments with adequate explanations of psychometric properties have been reported. The Caring Behaviors Inventory for Elders (Wolf, Goldberg, Crothers, & Jacobson, 2006) was developed to measure caring from the point of view of elders and their caregivers. In a convenient sample of 215 elders and 138 nurses from independent and assisted-living facilities, combined internal consistency was reported as .936. Five factors emerged from the data: attending to individual needs, showing respect, practicing knowledgeably and skillfully, respecting autonomy, and supporting religious/spiritual needs. The final 28-item instrument, limited by the convenient sample of elders and caregivers, has utility in this restricted population. The Caring Nurse–Patient Interaction Scale (Short Scale) of Cossette, Côté, Pepin, Ricard, and D'Aoust (2006) used 377 baccalaureate students from one school to explore attitudes and behaviors associated with caring. Four factors, namely relational care, clinical care, comforting care, and humanistic care, emerged with a 23-item solution. Internal consistency reliability varied from .61 to .94. A follow-up study (Cossette, Pepin, Côté, Poulin de Courval, 2008) confirmed the four factors in a group of 531 baccalaureate students.

The Caring Assessment Tool (CAT) is a 36-item instrument designed to capture patients' perceptions of nurse caring (Duffy, Hoskins, & Seifert, 2007). In an exploratory factor analysis of 557 patients from 5 acute care institutions, the tool performed well (alpha = .96), and 8 independent factors emerged from the data, all with appropriate internal consistency reliability (.757–.917). This tool was limited by the convenient sample, but it partially supported Watson's (1979, 1985) theory of human caring and is consistent with other empirical evidence. It is available in English, Spanish, and Japanese and offers nursing a caring instrument with little burden to patients.

Although a growing knowledge base regarding the measurement of caring is emerging, there continue to be issues related to the conceptual base of the instruments, adequate psychometrics, and the perspective of the evaluator. With regard to the latter factor, the recipient of caring (most often the patient) is the most direct source of caring knowledge. When measuring caring in clinical situations, the patient's perspective is always the most advantageous because patients' and nurses' perceptions of caring have been known to differ (Swanson, 1999). Likewise, when measuring caring among nursing students, families or caregivers, or nurses themselves, it is important to collect the data from those being "cared for."

Evaluating Caring Practice

Although measuring caring refers to quantifying the concept and is most often linked to research, *evaluation* of caring refers to using measurements to make judgments about caring (Oermann & Gaberson, 2006). Generally, evaluation requires a process designed to help reach conclusions about students, employees, programs, or services on the attainment of certain objectives or behaviors. Measurement is inherent in evaluation because criteria are identified, quantified, and assessed according to some scale in order to make decisions. Evaluation processes provide the basis for performance reviews, continuation or revisions of programs, and improvements in services. Data are collected, both ongoing (formative) or at the conclusion (summative), and are used to make informed decisions.

Because caring practice is founded on a set of beliefs or a philosophy of caring, it is important when evaluating professional performance to first articulate the knowledge, behaviors, and attitudes that define caring practice. The caring factors can help in this regard because they provide practical guidance on "how to care." (See Chapter 8 for some examples of staff-nurse competencies based on the Quality-Caring Model©.) In the context of a caring relationship, a student or employee can use the document together with a supervisor to actively participate and listen to suggestions on how to improve clinical practice. Such appraisals should be both ongoing and summative to stimulate reflection and improvement in caring practice.

Ideally, students and employees whose practice is based on caring will take an active role in evaluating that practice because the underlying relationship to the self is an important aspect of caring practice. The clinician who is "in touch" with him/herself will reflect in an ongoing pattern about the nature of the practice and how it can be advanced. The caring supervisor will observe, dialogue, provide ongoing feedback, identify strengths and challenges, and offer supportive guidance in an effort to assist the clinician to enhance his/her practice.

Evaluation of caring programs such as caring demonstration projects or a caring professional practice model requires a rigorous examination of its intended outcomes. Unfortunately, well-designed evaluations are often left undone because perceived complexity of the process, including the collection of data while simultaneously maintaining the program, seems daunting. Health care professionals, in particular, seem to rely on patients' comments or their own passion and feelings to conclude that a particular program or service is worthwhile. However, without proper evaluation, the value or usefulness of programs or services to patients and professionals is not known. An evaluation model provides a framework to guide the process. In the context of caring professional practice, the Quality-Caring Model provides a holistic and participatory model to guide program evaluation.

Using this model, structural components of program evaluation include characteristics of the participants. In this case, patients, providers, or organizational demographic data provide important information that may impact the processes or outcomes of a program and need to be captured. For example, patients who are more severely ill or have multiple comorbidities may influence how professional nurses use the caring factors and what outcomes can be realistically attained. Likewise, nurses with certain credentials (i.e., education, certifications) may provide care that varies from their peers—this may impact the results. And organizations who use specific staffing models or who provide more educational opportunities for professional nurses may inadvertently impact the processes and outcomes of care. Taking these factors into consideration during program evaluation allows one to modify the resulting data, lending credibility to the outcomes.

Process-based elements help individuals understand *how* their program is working. This is useful when staff and patients' opinions about a program or service are solicited in order to make adjustments, recommendations for improvement, or decisions about continuation. In one large demonstration project, for example, patients' perceptions of nurse caring behaviors (a process indicator) were used to make revisions to how a professional practice model was being implemented (Duffy, Baldwin, & Mastorovich, 2007). In this same project, nurses' feedback about the model implementation process was obtained through focus groups and was used to suggest ways to improve the practice. Identification of strengths and weaknesses in programs and services in order to streamline or adjust their delivery adds to effectiveness and efficiency.

One innovative project, the International Caring Comparative Database (ICCD) (Duffy, 2008), is a dynamic repository that began as a scholarly endeavor associated with the International Caritas Consortium, a part of the larger Watson Caring Science Institute (2008). This group of health professionals and institutions is connected through the use of caring theory in clinical, practice, and research projects. The ICCD is an open and flexible database that collects and evaluates patients' perceptions of nurse caring behaviors from health care institutions throughout the world. It stores the nursing-sensitive *process* indicator, nurse caring behaviors. This indicator of caring provides participating institutions with timely information about the processes of caring (from the patient's point of view). Regularly assessing caring processes allows clinicians and administrators to monitor improvements in nursing practice, to link caring processes with nursing-sensitive outcomes measures, to study ways that structural indicators such as staffing patterns or nurse credentials affect caring processes, and to examine trends over time. Using the CAT version IV and patient descriptors (e.g., age, gender, educational level), participating institutions receive unit-level comparative data reports to use for benchmarking, seeking out best practices, quality improvement, and research (Duffy, Hoskins, et al., 2007).

The ICCD is the only comparative database of caring behaviors performed by nurses. It has grown from an idea to a reality because health care institutions that use caring professional practice models as a foundation for nursing practice are actively seeking ways to connect and improve their services. Other *process* indicators, such as nurse manager caring behaviors and nurse educator caring behaviors, may be added in the future. (See Table 9.2 for information on how to participate in the ICCD.)

To validate, improve, or increase the impact of a program or service to patients or staff, *outcomes evaluation* is used. Outcomes evaluation

Table 9.2

PROCESS FOR PARTICIPATION IN THE INTERNATIONAL CARING COMPARATIVE DATABASE (ICCD)©

1. Agree to become a participant for one year.[a] Agency personnel involved in data collection/submission agree to complete a one-hour class (free to participants) in data collection and/or data entry. This class may be online or through a conference call or DVDs—no travel is required!

2. Appoint someone to serve as a liaison/contact person/site coordinator between your institution and the ICCD—complete a data form (to be determined) with an e-mail address for correspondence. The liaison/contact person/site coordinator will be responsible for data collection and submission and be available to answer questions from ICCD. He/she will also receive and disseminate quarterly reports from ICCD.

3. Identify data collectors on each unit/department—negotiate their commitment to quarterly data collection (excellent activity for those wishing to "climb" the clinical ladder or further their education).

4. Submit data according to the quarterly schedule[b] using the recommended format.[c]

5. On a quarterly basis, randomly select 10 percent of patients on each unit/department using a caring practice model; administer a one-page demographic form and the CAT version IV (attached and free to participants). It is recommended that patients selected be hospitalized for at least 24 hours prior to data collection to ensure that interaction with registered nurses has occurred. Collect all completed instruments, enter results in the recommended format, and send the data file to ICCD by the due date. For example, on a 30-bed unit, 3 patients would need to complete the instrument/s.

6. Promptly notify the Principal Investigator at ICCD if institution is no longer able to continue participation.

IN EXCHANGE FOR PARTICIPATION, ICCD WILL:

1. Assure anonymity and confidentiality of participant's institution, staff, and patients including presentations and publications of ICCD aggregated data.

2. Assure standards for data management including data integrity and data security.

3. Provide participants with quarterly reports including trends and comparisons to other institutions in the database. The reports will be provided to participants directly by ICCD. Provide updates to Caring Consortium semiannually.

(Continued)

Table 9.2

PROCESS FOR PARTICIPATION IN THE INTERNATIONAL CARING COMPARATIVE DATABASE (ICCD)© (Continued)

IN EXCHANGE FOR PARTICIPATION, ICCD WILL:

4. Assure that participants will have the opportunity to provide feedback to ICCD to guide future projects/opportunities.

5. Facilitate participants' publication/presentation desires through assistance as needed.

From *Participating Institution's Statement of Agreement*, by J. Duffy, 2008. Indianapolis: Indiana University.
[a]A fee schedule is necessary to clean, analyze, interpret, and create reports.
[b]September 30, December 31, March 31, June 30. [c]Web-based, user-entered.

includes identifying intended outcomes, prioritizing them, specifying measures or indicators of achievement, establishing criteria or targets (the number required) for success, collecting the information, and reporting the results (Meisenheimer, 1997). Indicators can be both quantitative (e.g., established instruments) or qualitative (e.g., observations, focus groups). Reporting the results of outcomes evaluation (especially to those providing the services) provides valuable information about what has been learned about the program or service. Both positive and negative results should always be reported in a format consistent with the audience. Using the outcomes, project directors can assess their attainment and the level of improvement and benchmark their results to other organizations. (See Table 9.3 for an example of the components used in a comprehensive evaluation of a caring demonstration project.)

Another aspect of program evaluation important to health care administrators in particular is the cost-benefit evaluation. This form of analysis contrasts alternatives and helps to determine the relative worth of programs or services. Comparisons to other programs can be useful when budgets are slim to help administrators make decisions about which programs to retain or let go. Insurers, funding agencies, and policymakers also need evaluation data to make decisions about continuation of programs. Finally, evaluation data can be used for public relations or marketing purposes to provide potential customers with important information about programs.

Table 9.3

EVALUATION MODEL FOR THE RELATIONSHIP-CENTERED CARING IN ACUTE CARE PROJECT

STRUCTURE	PROCESS	OUTCOMES
Patient	Patients' perceptions of nurse caring	Patient satisfaction
Age	Patients' perceptions of nursing responsiveness	Functional ability
Acuity	Patients' perceptions of	Pain
# Comorbidities	familiarity with the health care team	Falls
		Pressure ulcers
		Med errors
Nurse		
Age	Nurses' perceptions of	Vacancy rates
Education	work environment	Retention
Years experience		Satisfaction
System		
Nursing HPPD	Nursing time spent "in relationship"	Length of stay
		Readmission rates

(Duffy, 2005–2010). *Relationship-centered caring in acute care.* U.S. Health Resources and Services Administration #D66HPO5242-01-00.

RESEARCHING CARING

Studying the phenomenon of caring is difficult; yet, as an emerging profession, knowledge development in its core processes is necessary to advance nursing. Early qualitative methods were used to describe caring's attributes, to contrast caring and noncaring nursing situations (Reiman, 1986), to describe the importance of nurse caring in specific patient populations (Larson, 1984), and to learn more about nurse–patient relationships (Halldorsdottir, 1991). A recent metasynthesis of caring in nursing used 49 qualitative reports to better understand the concept (Finfgeld-Connett, 2008). Findings referred to caring as a context-specific interpersonal process performed by expert nurses in a working environment conducive to caring.

Swanson (1999) completed an excellent review of qualitative and quantitative caring knowledge and classified it in one of five levels:

the capacity for caring, concerns/commitments, conditions for caring, caring actions, and caring consequences. In this literary review, many studies focused on the nurse's capacity for caring, including several ethical studies. Conditions that affect caring, both nurse-related and organization-related, were described, as were some caring instruments. "Quantitative findings about the consequences of caring were minimal" (p. 52); however, coping and decreased psychological distress (Latham, 1996), increased patient satisfaction (Duffy, 1992), and increased nursing job satisfaction (Duffy, 1993) were found to be linked to caring. Swanson described most of the knowledge generated from studying caring as interpretive and urged researchers to build on this work to create practical measures and trial interventions using generalizable research designs.

Smith (2004) reviewed research using Watson's theory of caring and found 40 studies from 1988 to 2003 showing a sustained trajectory. They fell into the categories of the nature of nurse caring, nurse-caring behaviors as perceived by clients and nurses, human experiences and caring needs, and evaluating outcomes of caring in nursing practice and education. In addition, five instruments based on Watson's model were reported. Smith commented on the growing international interest in caring research, the diversity of designs, and the incongruence between nurse and patient perceptions of caring. She suggested several weaknesses in the research, including the lag behind Watson's newly evolved theory and the vagueness between findings and the theory, and urged future researchers to build on past strengths and address current gaps to move toward greater knowledge of caring.

Since that time, more study has been devoted to linking caring with patient outcomes, suggesting that nurse caring is a valuable aspect of health care that may impact patient satisfaction (Wolf et al., 1998), postoperative recovery (Swan, 1998), and anxiety (Burt, 2007). In the last study, Burt (2007) used the Quality-Caring Model to study the association between hospitalized older adults' perceptions of caring and selected outcomes of care. Using a random selection process of 84 hospitalized medical patients and controlling for gender, she found that caring explained 20.2% of the variance in anxiety ($p < .01$).

Factor analytic work has served to identify several robust dimensions that make up caring (Cossette et al., 2006, 2008; Duffy, Hoskins, et al., 2007; Wolf et al., 2006), but limited caring intervention studies have been completed. Smith, Kemp, Hemphill, and Vojir (2002) used Watson's (1979, 1985) and Rogers's (1970) models to test the use of therapeutic massage in hospitalized cancer patients. Using two groups (N = 41), they found pain, sleep quality, symptom distress, and anxiety improved from baseline in those patients who received the intervention. Erci and colleagues (2003) used Watson's theory to test the effectiveness of a caring relationship on blood pressure and quality of life in hypertensive patients in Turkey. Using a one-group pre/posttest design with a sample of 52 hypertensive patients, they found significant differences in blood pressure (decreased) and quality of life (increased) posttesting. Although limited in design due to lack of controls, the attempt to demonstrate the effect of caring relationships on outcomes in a specific patient population is impressive.

Using the Quality-Caring Model as the foundation, Duffy, Hoskins, and Dudley-Brown (2005) developed a caring intervention to test its effects on outcomes of community-dwelling older adults with heart failure. Using a comprehensive telephone-mediated intervention that emphasized a consistent nurse (in the context of a caring patient–nurse relationship) and dedicated time for symptom monitoring, education, and emotional support, the team designed a protocol for testing in a randomized clinical trial. (See Figure 9.1 for the research model.) The final sample size (N = 32) was too small to detect significant differences, yet reduced readmissions and increased patient satisfaction and quality of life were reported in the intervention group (Duffy & Hoskins, in press). Finally, Swanson's Caring Interventions for Couples Who Have Miscarried randomized clinical trial used four groups to test behavioral, self-caring among couples and a combined behavioral and self-caring intervention on well-being in couples who have miscarried (National Institutes of Health, 2008). The study used Swanson's middle-range theory of caring (1991), and the study variables were measured longitudinally. To expand the knowledge base of caring, however, the need continues for rigorous research approaches using sophisticated methods. Such research should build on the work of others, extend over time, and be completed in varied populations. Furthermore, explicitly establishing the congruence between the research variables and caring conceptual models will serve to advance caring-specific theory.

ADVANCING THE SCIENCE OF CARING

To extend the understanding and strengthen the evidence of caring (specifically nurse caring) as a significant variable in the health care

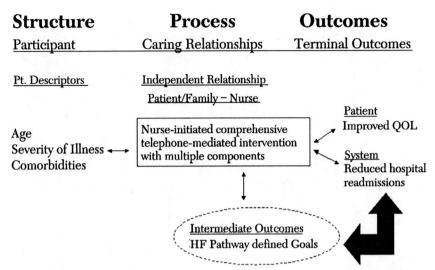

Figure 9.1 Research model guiding the study Outcomes of Telehealth and Homecare in Heart Failure. Supported by a grant from the National Institute of Nursing Research #NR 008005-01A1 and The Catholic University of America, Washington, D.C.

process, much more research must be conducted and disseminated. A caring research model may provide the framework for advancing the science (see Figure 9.2).

First, identifying research priorities might be a task for national/international organizations, such as the International Association for Human Caring (IAHC), or schools of nursing, foundations, or even individual researchers. Second, continuing to build on the foundation of caring science using multiple methods will enrich the knowledge base. Refining existing measures of caring using appropriate conceptual definitions and adequate psychometric properties, with particular emphasis on the patient's view, will allow for correlational studies and multisite comparisons. Qualitative studies permitting in-depth assessment of caring relationships including the lived experiences of all members, culturally based caring, the complexities of caring relationships, how caring capacity develops, and requirements for caring relationships are necessary. Using approaches such as observation, interviews, focus groups, narratives, and other interpretive methods will enrich the science. Quantitative methods linking caring to specific patient, nurse, and system outcomes will strengthen the evidence regarding the value of caring in clinical practice. Likewise, linking faculty caring to student learning outcomes and administrative caring to healthy work environments

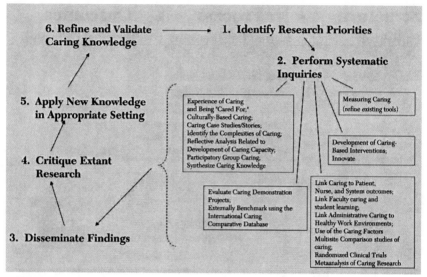

Figure 9.2 Model for advancing caring science.

for professional nurses will provide the basis for innovation in these settings.

Developing caring-based interventions for testing in quantitative studies is necessary to provide high levels of evidence for caring-based nursing practice and to validate caring theory. Caring-based interventions are complicated to design because little has been done in this area, and practical limitations for testing can be challenging. Nevertheless, caring-based interventions must be trialed to better understand how they contribute to health care outcomes. Choosing a caring-based conceptual framework to support the intervention followed by an application based on prior research and organized to meet the needs of the population under study is paramount. Developing a protocol describing the content, strength, and frequency of the intervention allows for replication. Using probability sampling and longitudinal studies, questions such as what is the effect of the intervention on specific outcomes of care can be answered. Integrating cost-effectiveness components will add to the understanding of the intervention's worth.

The National Institutes of Nursing Research (NINR) has designated several areas of clinical research emphasis that may provide suggestions for future caring clinical research (NINR, 2007). Promoting health and preventing disease is an area that seeks to understand factors and decision making that influence health behaviors and uses interventions to increase such behaviors over time. Caring-based interventions could be designed for specific populations geared toward health promotion. For example, in school-age children, reducing the threats related to obesity might be eased through targeted interventions provided in the context of caring relationships with school nurses or counselors. Or, increasing regular exercise among elderly women living in assisted-living facilities might be tested using a walking group with consistent caring nurses.

The second NINR clinical research priority is improving quality of life. In populations at risk or with chronic disease, increasing self-caring behaviors contributes positively to quality of life. Self-caring, rather that self-management, is a combination of using the inner awareness and resources of the self together with externally focused assistance by a dedicated health care professional in the context of a caring relationship. Self-caring builds on a person's strengths and uses positive thoughts or intentions to accept encouragement and assistance from others (when necessary), to adopt healthy behaviors and maintain independence. Caring-based interventions that seek to increase self-caring or studies that identify factors associated with self-caring practices are warranted. How self-caring impacts quality of life or maintenance of independence, especially in those with chronic illnesses, is important.

The management of symptoms, the third NINR research emphasis area, can be augmented by caring studies that use holistic approaches toward symptom management. Nonpharmacologic interventions, such as optimizing sleep patterns, frequent reorientation, decreasing environmental triggers, massage, family engagement, healing aesthetics, and individualized comfort measures provided in the context of caring relationships, are examples of holistic approaches. Identifying barriers to symptom management, using quasi and experimental designs focused on patient-defined comfort, and using qualitative methods to elicit lived experiences or culturally congruent ideas related to symptom management will meet this mandate.

The rise in chronic disease has increased the need to better understand caregiver needs. Questions such as: Do caring relationships with health care providers improve self-caring and quality of life among caregivers? or How well does a caregiver–care recipient relationship sustain time? are important to answer. Caring-based interventions for caregivers and demonstration projects that honor the importance of caregivers to the health of those with chronic illnesses are issues of deep concern for nursing.

Decreasing health disparities by meeting the caring needs of underserved populations or testing culturally congruent caring interventions is also desperately needed. Finally, studying caring end-of-life interventions based on patient preferences would provide evidence of nursing's value in this vulnerable population.

In education, the National League for Nursing (NLN) has outlined innovations, educational evaluation, and evidence-based reform as research priorities (NLN, 2008). The impact of caring-based pedagogies on student learning, how caring relationships are best learned in simulated-teaching environments, the student–teacher relationship, clinical teaching, and preparation of nurse faculty for teaching caring relationships as the basis for professional practice are research questions that would enhance the educational environment and possibly student learning.

Program evaluation including student satisfaction and evaluation (including grading and testing) of student caring practice/s would provide evidence of caring competence upon graduation. Important to the discussion of caring educational research is the preparation of the next generation of nurse scientists. Without role models conducting caring research in schools of nursing, graduate students will not get the chance to participate in advancing caring science. Nurse researchers involved in caring research must involve students at all levels in their research, explain their methods and results during class discussions, invite participation in specific projects, demonstrate the consistency between caring conceptual frameworks and specific research variables, and model the process of caring research.

Similarly, those in leadership positions should take seriously the benefits of carefully evaluating caring programs and services as well as conducting research. The American Organization for Nurse Executives' (AONE; 2005) Institute for Patient Care Research & Education provides seed money to fund small studies about leadership, excellence in patient care, and health policy. And, the U.S. Health Resources and Services Administration (HRSA) offers funding under the mechanism Nurse Education, Practice, and Retention Program (NEPR), more specifically, the retention objective: enhancing patient care delivery systems (U.S. Department of Health and Human Services, 2007). Demonstration projects using caring-based professional practice models, benchmarking caring practices among multiple sites, evaluating the impact of healing environments on nurse satisfaction and retention, and enhancing interprofessional caring will add to the growing science of caring.

Using strategies such as interprofessional teams, applying tools where data are pooled from multiple sites, and integrating biological, behavioral, and cost-effectiveness methods will eventually enable us to make predictions about how nurses with certain characteristics will perform the caring factors, the proper "dose" of caring for particular patient populations, the most effective ways to learn caring, and the relative worth of caring practices. As Quinn, Smith, Ritenbaugh, Swanson, and Watson (2003) emphasize, there are several cogent reasons for studying caring relationships. Among them are: It provides a rationale for improving care; it may expose the significant role of the nurse in healing and help ease the nursing shortage; and it will help validate or reject existing theory. Based on this justification, nurse researchers have a social responsibility to study caring in nursing.

The third aspect of the research model depicted in Figure 9.2 is dissemination. Relevant manuscripts and doctoral dissertations published in high-quality journals will expose others to caring research. Likewise, presentations at professional organizations and using the results of caring studies to create or revise existing policy add to the science.

Through the daily application of evidence-based practice, critically appraising caring research is important to judge the trustworthiness of study findings and to translate credible results to the bedside. Applying new knowledge in the appropriate setting may help to transform the work environment for nurses such that they find meaning in the important work they do. Finally, drawing conclusions from research about caring theory helps to validate and refine it.

Explicitly stating the caring theory that undergirds research studies adds valuable knowledge for the profession and provides the basis for future nursing care (Fawcett, 2008).

SUMMARY

Measuring caring through well-designed and effectively applied instruments is crucial to advancing caring science. Criteria for judging caring instruments are presented along with a discussion of the conceptual basis for caring and the unique perspective of the recipient of caring. Reaching conclusions, or evaluating caring practice, learning, or programs is reviewed through the lens of the Quality-Caring Model. Research on caring is considered, including several recent studies, but emphasis is placed on advancing the science of caring through an organized research model that calls for multiple methods and approaches. Identifying research priorities, building on the existing caring research, and developing caring-based interventions combined with advanced investigational strategies will eventually enable predictions and validate caring theory. Dissemination of results and quickly translating credible findings to practice environments provide encouragement for the future of nursing.

CALLS TO ACTION

When it is necessary to identify the presence or absence of caring, determine the frequency of its occurrence, its appropriateness or importance, its link to other variables, explain differences among groups and individuals' opinions of it, and determine if caring should be measured. **Brainstorm** ways to best assess caring.

Despite the fact that multiple tools exist that purport to measure caring, concerns linger about what conceptual base was used to develop items, the adequacy of psychometric properties, and from whose perspective the information is obtained. **Compare** caring instruments for use in your work.

A caring supervisor/faculty member is key to assisting students and employees to evaluate their practice. Through observation, ongoing exchanges including regular feedback, confirming strengths and pointing out challenges, and providing reassurance and sup-

(continued)

portive guidance, the supervisor can assist the clinician to improve his/her practice. Students and employees whose practice is based on caring and whose underlying relationship to the self is part of this practice should accept the supervisor's input and use it to progress. Clinicians who are "in touch" with themselves will integrate supervisory feedback with their knowledge of self to advance their practice and expand their own lives. **Learn** more about your employees' or students' caring behaviors; **welcome** feedback about your practice from your supervisor.

A thorough assessment of caring programs, such as caring demonstration projects or caring professional practice models, rests on the appraisal of their intended outcomes. **Estimate** the value added to your organization from the caring practice of professional nurses.

More research is necessary to extend the understanding and strengthen the evidence of caring (specifically nurse caring) as a significant variable in the health care process. **Select** a research question using caring as a variable.

A devoted health care professional who provides help and support in the context of a caring relationship together with the inner awareness and reserves of strength found in the self generates self-caring, a renewable energy source that leads to a small individual change. Many small individual changes, however, expand over time to large system changes. **Go to** the International Association of Human Caring at (http://www.humancaring.org) to get more information about human caring.

Potential research investigations appropriate to the educational environment include: the impact of caring-based pedagogies on student learning, how caring relationships are best learned in simulated teaching environments, the nature of student–teacher relationships, clinical teaching using caring as a foundation, and preparation of nurse faculty for teaching-caring relationships as the basis for professional practice. **Encourage** a nursing colleague in the investigation of caring pedagogies.

(continued)

Important professional knowledge is advanced by overtly stating the caring theory that undergirds research studies. Such knowledge will provide the empirical evidence for expert nursing care. **Study** at least two caring theories.

Reflective Questions/Applications for Students

1. Discuss the term *measurement* as it applies to caring relationships. Is measurement of caring a priority for nursing? Why or why not?
2. Contrast qualitative and quantitative research methods. What are the pros and cons of each as they relate to caring relationships?
3. Develop three research questions based on caring. What will you do with these questions? How might you participate in such studies?
4. Using the criteria for evaluating caring instruments (Table 9.1), select three caring instruments and appraise them. Which one would be the most appropriate to your situation?
5. Differentiate among the terms *measurement, evaluation,* and *research.*
6. Using the Quality-Caring Model, develop an evaluation plan for a program you are interested in. Identify *structure, process,* and *outcomes* elements that would be appropriate, and discuss the tools, methods for data collection, and how results will be disseminated to make decisions about continuing the program.
7. Using appropriate appraisal techniques, critique one qualitative and one quantitative caring study. Are the results credible? Would you adopt them in practice? Why or why not?

Reflective Questions/Applications for Educators

8. Identify three caring research priorities. What research questions do you suggest? Elaborate on the methods you would employ to answer each of the questions.
9. As a faculty member with research responsibilities, what approach would you use to encourage the design of innovative caring-based interventions at your institution?

10. Using the caring research model depicted in Figure 9.2, identify three research priority areas.
11. As an educator, how might you encourage others to innovate and/or participate in demonstration projects that emphasize caring relationships? Be specific.
12. Develop a caring-based intervention for a population of interest. Make sure you include the frequency, the location, and the appropriate "dose" for the intervention.
13. Design a study to examine the impact of self-caring on the quality of life for chronically ill diabetic persons.
14. Design a study to assess the impact of caring-based pedagogies on student learning.

Reflective Questions/Applications for Nurse Leaders

15. Describe the mechanism for employee evaluation in your organization. Are caring behaviors explicitly stated? Is active participation by the employee an essential component? What recommendations do you have to improve the process?
16. Analyze the advantages and disadvantages of the International Comparative Database for your organization.
17. Discuss how you would go about partnering with a school of nursing to pilot a caring demonstration project.

REFERENCES

American Organization for Nurse Executives. (2005). Retrieved December 1, 2007, from http://www.aone.org/aone/institute/seedgrant.html

Baumann, S. (2003). Caring science and the development of measurement approaches. *Nursing Science Quarterly, 16,* 353–355.

Beck, C. T. (1999). Quantitative measurement of caring. *Journal of Advanced Nursing, 30*(1), 24–32.

Boykin, A., & Schoenhofer, S. (1993). *Nursing as caring: A model for transforming practice.* New York: National League for Nursing.

Burns, N., & Grove, S. K. (2005). *The practice of nursing research: Conduct, critique, utilization* (5th ed.). St. Louis, MO: Elsevier Saunders.

Burt, K. (2007). The relationship between nurse caring and selected outcomes of care in hospitalized older adults. *Dissertation Abstracts International* (UMI No. 3257620).

Cossette, S., Côté, J. K., Pepin, J., Ricard, N., & D'Aoust, L. X. (2006). A dimensional structure of nurse-patient interactions from a caring perspective: Refinement of the Caring Nurse-Patient Interaction Scale (CNPI-Short Scale). *Journal of Advanced Nursing, 55*(2), 198–214.

Cossette, S., Pepin, J., Côté, J. K., & Poulin de Courval, F. (2008). The multidimensionality of caring: A confirmatory factor analysis of the Caring Nurse-Patient Interaction Short Scale. *Journal of Advanced Nursing, 61*(6), 699–710.

Duffy, J. (1992). Impact of nurse caring on patient outcomes. In D. A. Gaut (Ed.), *The presence of caring in nursing* (pp. 113–136). New York: National League for Nursing

Duffy, J. (1993). Caring behaviors of nurse managers: Relationships to staff nurse satisfaction and retention. In D. Gaut (Ed.), *A global agenda for caring* (pp. 365–377). New York: National League for Nursing.

Duffy, J. (2008). *International Caring Comparative Database. Participating Institution's Statement of Agreement.* Indianapolis, IN: Indiana University Press.

Duffy, J., Baldwin, J., & Mastorovich, M. J. (2007). Using the Quality-Caring Model to organize patient care delivery. *Journal of Nursing Administration, 37*(12), 546–551.

Duffy, J., & Hoskins, L. M. (in press). Improvements in readmission and quality of life following a caring-based nursing intervention. *Journal of Nursing Care Quality.*

Duffy, J., Hoskins, L. M., & Dudley-Brown, S. (2005). Development and testing of a caring-based intervention for older adults with heart failure. *Journal of Cardiovascular Nursing, 20*(5), 325–333.

Duffy, J., Hoskins, L. M., & Seifert, R. F. (2007). Dimensions of caring: Psychometric properties of the caring assessment tool. *Advances in Nursing Science, 30*(3), 235–245.

Erci, B., Sayan, A., Tortumluog-lu, G., Kiliç, D., Sahin, O., & Gungurmus, Z. (2003). The effectiveness of Watson's Caring Model on the quality of life and blood pressure of patients with hypertension. *Journal of Advanced Nursing, 41*(2), 130–139.

Fawcett, J. (2008). The added value of nursing conceptual-model-based research. *Journal of Advanced Nursing, 61*(6), 583.

Finfgeld-Connett, D. (2008). Meta-synthesis of caring in nursing. *Journal of Clinical Nursing, 17,* 196–204.

Halldorsdottir, S. (1991). Five basic modes of being with another. In D. Gaut & M. M. Leininger (Eds.), *Caring: The compassionate healer* (pp. 37–49). New York: National League for Nursing.

Larson, P. J. (1984). Important nurse caring behaviors perceived by patients with cancer. *Oncology Nursing Forum, 11*(6), 46–50.

Latham, C. (1996). Predictors of patient outcomes following interactions with nurses. *Western Journal of Nursing Research, 18*(5), 548–564.

Leininger, M. M. (1981). The phenomenon of caring: Importance of research and theoretical considerations. In M. M. Leininger (Ed.), *Caring: An essential human need.* Thorofare, NJ: Slack.

Meisenheimer, C. G. (1997). *Improving quality: A guide to effective programs.* Boston, MA: Jones and Bartlett Publishers.

National Institute of Nursing Research (NINR). (2007, August 14). Retrieved March 16, 2008, from http://www.ninr.nih.gov/NR/rdonlyres/F85C02CA-1EE3-40F7-BDA4-3901F2284E96/0/StrategicAreasofResearchEmphasis.pdf

National Institutes of Health. (2008). *Couples' miscarriage healing project: Randomized trial.* Retrieved March 13, 2008, from http://clinicaltrials.gov/ct2/show/NCT00194844

National League for Nursing (NLN). (2008). *Research priorities in nursing education.* Retrieved April 2, 2008, from http://www.nln.org/research/priorities.htm

Oermann, M. H., & Gaberson, K. B. (2006). *Evaluation and testing in nursing education.* New York: Springer Publishing.

Quinn, J., Smith, M., Ritenbaugh, C., Swanson, K., & Watson, J. (2003). Research guidelines for assessing the impact of the healing relationship in clinical nursing. *Alternative Therapies, 9*(3), A65–A79.

Reiman, D. J. (1986). Non-caring and caring in the clinical setting: Patients' descriptions. *Topics in Clinical Nursing, 8*(2), 30–36.

Roach, S. (1984). *Caring: The human mode of being: Implications for nursing—perspectives in caring* (Monograph 1). Toronto, CA: Faculty of Nursing, University of Toronto.

Rogers, M. E. (1970). *An introduction to the theoretical basis of nursing.* Philadelphia, PA: FA Davis.

Smith, M. (2004). Review of research related to Watson's theory of caring. *Nursing Science Quarterly, 17*(13), 13–25.

Smith, M. C., Kemp, J., Hemphill, L., & Vojir, C. P. (2002). Outcomes of therapeutic massage for hospitalized cancer patients. *Journal of Nursing Scholarship, 34*(3), 257–262.

Swan, B. (1998). Postoperative nursing care contributions to symptom distress and functional status after ambulatory surgery. *Medical Surgical Nursing, 7*(3), 148–158.

Swanson, K. (1991). Empirical development of a middle-range theory of caring. *Nursing Research, 40*(3), 161–166.

Swanson, K. M. (1999). What's known about caring in nursing: A literary meta-analysis. In A. S. Hinshaw, J. Shaver, & S. Feetham (Eds.), *Handbook of clinical nursing research* (pp. 31–60). Thousand Oaks, CA: Sage Publications.

U.S. Department of Health and Human Services. (2007). *Nurse Education, Practice and Retention (NEPR) program guidance* (HRSA-08-028). Rockville, MD: Health Resources and Services Administration, Bureau of Health Professions, Division of Nursing (CFDA), No. 93.359.

Watson, J. (1979). *Nursing: The philosophy and science of caring.* Boston: Little, Brown and Company.

Watson, J. (1985). *Nursing: Human science and human care.* Norwalk, CT: Appleton-Century-Crofts.

Watson, J. (2002). *Instruments for assessing and measuring caring in nursing and health sciences.* New York: Springer Publishing.

Watson Caring Science Institute. (2008). Retrieved August 24, 2008, from www.watson caringscience.org

Wolf, Z., Zuzelo, P., Goldberg, E., Crothers, R., & Jacobson, N. (2006). The caring behaviors inventory for elders: Development and psychometric characteristics. *International Journal for Human Caring, 10*(1), 49–59.

10

The Quality-Caring Model© Revisited

There are two ways of spreading light: to be the candle or the mirror that reflects it.

—Edith Wharton

Keywords: **nursing, future, quality caring**

ENVISIONING THE FUTURE

Many futurist authors have speculated on how people will live, work, die, be educated, and pay for and experience health care 50 years from now. In fact, the World Future Society (2008) specializes in predicting future phenomena, regularly publishes a magazine, and hosts an annual convention. In general, trends related to the rise of eastern nations as world powers, increasing innovation on the Internet, globalization, the human genome project, escalating epidemics (both acute and chronic), and the mushrooming age of the majority population have been cited as important determinants of the future (Canton, 2006). Others see more attention to the environment, "intelligent" machines (robots) that perform more mundane tasks, and nanotechnology and quantum computing allowing for increased computing power and improved drug delivery (Foresight Nanotech Institute, 2008). Actually, the National Nanotechnology Initiative (NNI) was established

189

in 2001 to coordinate the research and development work of scientists from many U.S. federal agencies (NNI, 2008). As one author contended, "when intelligence can be embodied in devices that are portable or implantable—they form intimate connections with the body—and become companions" (Benford & Malartre, 2007, p. 16).

Still others believe that violence, extremism, and security issues will dominate the culture, while a move away from organized religion to more individualized spirituality is the view from some religious and secular groups (Chopra, 2008; Heckel, 2008; Tippett, 2008).

While no one can predict the future with certainty, there are general trends that lend themselves to thinking about how one might be living beyond 2060. For example, the varying value of the dollar and the recent global credit problem render it plausible that other currencies may dominate purchasing power or living standards may be compromised. The continued rise in energy prices affecting most of the world's commodities will generate changes in automobile production, spur more telecommuting, and affect air travel and food production. As the years go by, food may actually rival oil as the driving economic force because the demand for food by the world's rising populations may outpace supply. A new or maybe a couple of new-generation Internets may evolve that offer higher speed and interactivity. New world superpower/s may create political tensions and affect national policy, while immigration pressures in the United States may ease. Related to education, much more distance and experiential offerings will dominate elementary and secondary programs. In fact, many more young students will learn at home and meet in groups during experiential and seminar formats. At the college level, distance learning is already a reality, and improved systems will allow students and faculty members to teach and learn from home while benefiting from worldwide experts. Discoveries related to space travel or ocean exploration will be inviting, but bringing them to market in a cost-effective manner will prove difficult. The acceptance of genetically enhanced foods and other controversial advancements will invite much discourse.

In health care, the United States will continue to see improved technological advances that will allow individuals to benefit from lab and diagnostic care at the point of service, and many of these will be offered over the counter. Advances in imaging and miniature or robotic devices for minimally invasive surgery will be used

(continued)

more frequently. Increasingly large integrated health medical record systems connecting physicians' offices to hospitals and outpatient clinics will provide the backbone for quality improvement activities. Patient-controlled medical records with smart cards or, as some have suggested, implanted computer chips will enable improved communication and coordination (Kondro, 2007; Neame, 1997). Genetic progress will advance the targeted drug therapies that have already started and allow at-home risk assessments that will personalize health care and profoundly change medicine (Ginsburg & McCarthy, 2001; Lanfear & McLeod, 2007). Most of these advances will have the capacity to make the human lifespan longer. This will bring with it the paradox of a longer life versus quality of life (Butler, 2008). And, as has been the case for many years, health care costs will continue to rise.

In 2007, total health care spending in the United States represented 16% of the gross domestic product (GDP). Total spending was $2.3 *trillion* in 2007, or $7,600 per person (Poisal et al., 2007). U.S. health care spending is expected to increase at similar levels for the next decade reaching $4.2 trillion in 2016, or 20% of GDP. Workers are now paying $1,400 more in premiums annually for family coverage than they did in 2000 (The Henry J. Kaiser Family Foundation, 2007). In spite of this, there remains disagreement among policy makers, health care providers, and the American public about the best way to address health care costs. These continuously escalating costs will severely compromise employers', individuals', and the federal government's ability to pay for health care. Based on the political climate of the future, some form of universal health insurance will likely cover Americans who will continue to become savvier about health care and voice their concerns about their own care. Participative decision-making between provider and patient will become more the rule rather than the exception. Emergency department overcrowding may decrease, but hospitals will see an even higher rise in acute illnesses, while chronic and less acute illnesses will be treated at home. Physicians will make virtual office visits, and professional nurses will monitor chronically ill or recovering surgical patients through telehealth approaches. And while these advances are encouraging, the challenges of increasing consumer participation in health care; older, more chronically ill patients and their caregivers; improving quality and reducing errors in health care; and preparing enough qualified health care providers will continue to challenge the system over the next few years. And the persistent problems inherent in professional nursing (e.g., shortages, workload, job satisfaction) will tax hard-working professional nurses if the same old solutions are applied.

The projected advances and challenges simultaneously affecting health care highlight the growing complexity of an integrated, interactive, interdependent, and global system that requires a more sophisticated workforce—one that understands the significance of big picture thinking; whose practice is based on knowledge, multiple, and oftentimes competing connections; and one that values relationships as the basis for actions and decision making. This new health care system is emerging rapidly, and the shift to such sweeping transformation is already occurring.

Big picture or systems thinking is a reflective, evaluative process that enables one to visualize the whole, focus on the interaction among many parts, and see where and how he/she contributes to it. It is an expanded view that raises understanding (or consciousness), allows one to notice his/her importance to the whole, gain more insight, and, in the case of nursing, actively create the desired outcome. Slowing down, making time, and reflecting contribute to systems thinking. Senge, in *The Fifth Discipline* (1990), spoke about the importance of systems thinking to individuals and the organizations in which they work.

Practice based on knowledge not only reflects systems thinking but is one of the hallmarks of a profession (Lusk, 1997), and in the case of nursing, Fawcett, Watson, Neuman, Hinton-Walker, and Fitzpatrick (2001) remind us of the link between nursing theory, inquiry, evidence, and practice. That link, when fully established, verifies the value or significance of a profession and distinguishes the influence or contributions it makes to society. A practice profession that *uses* the knowledge of relationships as the basis for its work understands the nature of humans as they exist in union with the universe. And a practice profession that acknowledges and acts in accordance with its implicit knowledge is able to progress and advance itself. These ideas have assisted in the redefinition of the Quality-Caring Model.

QUALITY CARING, REVISITED

The philosophical and theoretical underpinnings of the revised Quality-Caring Model continue to draw upon earlier works in quality (e.g., Donabedian, 1966) and nursing with particular emphasis on Nightingale (1992), King (1981), and Watson (1979). Various mid-range theories also inform the model, such as Irvine's Role Effectiveness Model (Irvine, Sidani, & McGillis Hall, 1998) and Swanson's middle-range Theory of Caring (1991). With regard to the term *quality,* it remains nonlinear and continuous in nature and is associated with words such as knowledge, learning, innovation, and improvement. It is now more often referred to as a science with specialized evaluative processes (Berwick, 2008). And the most important aspect of quality is the understanding that it is a never-ending quest for excellence that is an intrinsic part of everyone's job in health care (Batalden & Davidoff, 2007). This definition implies that nurses, *all nurses,* are continuously involved in improving their practice, including the parts of it that interact with other health care providers. Active engagement in knowledge-generation through research, innovation, or improvement activities helps one learn about him/herself, patients/families/caregivers, and the health care system and then use that knowledge to advance (see Figure 10.1).

In this way of building excellence, one learns continuously through all forms of research, clinical experience-generated knowing, and personal reflection (Antrobus, 1997). Practicing through the lens of constant learning becomes the norm, each patient becomes an experiment, and learning about the self contributes to practice. Most important is the notion of action or *using* the knowledge produced to advance practice by accelerating the way clinical knowledge is produced and quickly

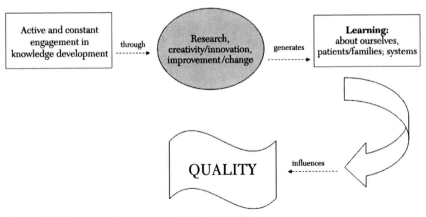

Figure 10.1 Learning through knowledge-generation.

converting statistical results into practice changes. One model for hastening learning, especially at the local level, is the Context/Mechanisms/ Outcomes (CMO) model (Pawson & Tilley, 1997). In this model, traditional randomized clinical trials and pre/posttesting are still used, but when improvements are needed or opportunities present themselves at a particular site, using the context (social and cultural conditions) and the most appropriate mechanisms (actual intervention or opportunity) for that site provide more practical findings that can be introduced easier. This approach (called practice-based evidence by some [Horn & Gassaway, 2007]) recognizes the knowledge of clinicians and often produces results more efficiently. Quality or excellence, then, can be said to be dynamic, fully integrated with practice, and scientific.

> Caring, on the other hand, is implicitly tied to *human beings* as they exist in relationship to each other, communities or groups, and the universe. Humans as multidimensional beings are worthy individuals who vary in terms of characteristics, unique experiences, beliefs, and attitudes. Using this variance, caring relationships enhance quality by bringing into play normal everyday human interactions that provide feedback about life experiences and human advancement.

The multidimensional nature of humans, when considered in its totality, constitutes a holistic perspective some call an energy field or phenomenal field and some religions call the soul (Watson, 1979). Ill persons have the added characteristic of severity, which denotes just how sick they are. Severity of illness is an important characteristic of ill persons because it impacts the processes and outcomes of health care (Sidani & Braden, 1998); as such, it must be accounted for in measures of quality. Humans interact in relationship with other beings and evolve over time and in the context of the larger universe. These connections actually sustain and enrich human existence. With adequate attention to the self, humans can blend external with internal ways of knowing to raise their consciousness or awareness. Finally, human beings live and work in communities or shared space where members are empowered through relationships to advance (see Figure 10.2). Active participation in one's community strengthens the health and quality of life of its members.

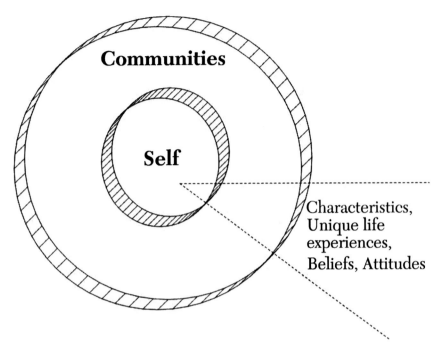

Figure 10.2 Multidimensional humans "in relationship" to themselves and their communities.

In health care situations, persons with health needs meet in relationship with health care providers who function independently and collaboratively with them. Independent relationships are those between patients and families and a health care provider, in this case, the professional nurse. Collaborative relationships are necessary to cohesively provide services such that they remain holistic and complementary. Such three-way encounters are *relationship-centered* when the health professionals work in unison and mutually partner with patients and families in the delivery of health care services (see Figure 10.3).

Furthermore, when the relationship is grounded in the caring factors, a human connection occurs that is transpersonal (more than the individuals alone) and results in a knowing of the other that anticipates, guides, provides for, teaches and learns, protects, and advocates. This form of relationship has the potential to be transforming for all involved. The caring factors, namely, *mutual problem-solving, attentive reassurance, human respect, encouraging manner, healing environment, appreciation of unique meanings, affiliation needs,* and *basic human needs,* are

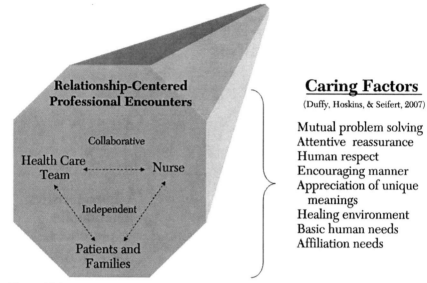

Figure 10.3 Relationship-centered professional encounters.

fundamental and unique to the revised Quality-Caring Model because, although derived from theory, they have been preliminarily validated (Duffy, Hoskins, & Seifert, 2007). These factors, when applied expertly and over time, lead to "feeling cared for" in the recipient. This reaction is a necessary antecedent to risk-taking, learning, follow-through, disclosure, and future interactions. Caring relationships with self, communities, patients and families, and between members of the health care team arouse persons', groups', and systems' capabilities to change, learn and develop, or self-advance. In other words, original, unique systems gradually advance through these multiple complex interactions; such systems, whether they are individual persons, groups of persons, or organizational systems, manifest as self-healing or self-caring. This growth is fueled by the caring energy shared among the participants (see Figure 10.4).

Self-advancing systems are *quality* systems in that they reflect dynamic positive progress that enhances the systems' well-being. This process is not linear but has highs and lows and emerges gradually over time and in space. It unifies the evidence and humanness required for excellence and transcends the current extremes of modernism and postmodernism.

Self-Advancing Systems

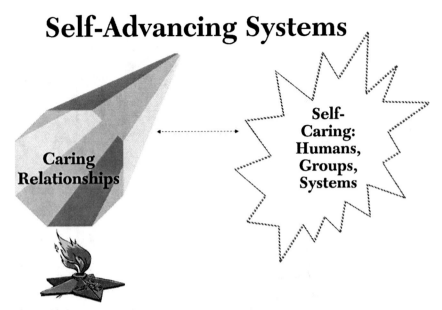

Figure 10.4 Self-advancing systems.

According to Roy (2000), "understanding human consciousness, awareness of self and environment, and accountability for the integration of human and environment creative processes is basic to envision and plan for the future" (p. 2). Caring relationships are crucial to this movement.

Assumptions of the revised Quality-Caring Model (see Figure 10.5) include the following:

Humans are multidimensional beings capable of growth and change.

Humans exist in relationship to themselves, others, communities or groups, nature (or the environment), and the universe.

Humans evolve over time and in space.

Humans are inherently worthy.

Caring is embedded in the daily work of nursing.

Caring is a tangible concept that can be measured.

Caring relationships benefit both the carer and the one being cared for.

Caring relationships benefit society.

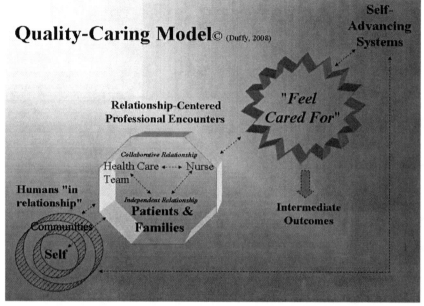

Figure 10.5 Revised Quality-Caring Model©.

Caring is done "in relationship."

Feeling "cared for" is a positive emotion.

Propositions from the revised Quality-Caring Model include:

Human caring capacity can be developed.

Caring relationships are composed of discrete factors.

Caring relationships require intent, specialized knowledge, and time.

Engagement in communities through caring relationships enhances self-caring.

Independent caring relationships between patients and nurses influence feeling "cared for."

Collaborative caring relationships among nurses and members of the health care team influence feeling "cared for."

Feeling "cared for" is an antecedent to self-advancing systems.

Feeling "cared for" influences the attainment of intermediate and terminal health outcomes.

Self-advancement is a nonlinear, complex process that emerges over time and in space.

Self-advancing systems are naturally self-caring or self-healing.

Relationships characterized as caring contribute to individual, group, and system self-advancement.

> The overall role of the nurse in this model is to engage in caring relationships with self and others to engender feeling "cared for." Such actions positively influence intermediate and terminal health outcomes, including those that are nursing-sensitive. Feeling "cared for" assists patients and families to assume self-healing or self-caring ways.

Specific responsibilities of the professional nurse include:

Attain and continuously advance knowledge and expertise in the caring factors.

Initiate, cultivate, and sustain caring relationships with patients and families.

Initiate, cultivate, and sustain caring relationships with other nurses and all members of the health care team.

Maintain an awareness of the patient/family point of view.

Carry on self-caring activities, including personal and professional development.

Integrate caring relationships with specific evidenced-based nursing interventions to positively influence health.

Advance quality health care through research and continuous improvement.

Using the expertise of caring relationships embedded in nursing, actively participate in community groups.

Contribute to the knowledge of caring and, ultimately, the profession of nursing using all forms of knowing.

Maintain an open, flexible approach.

QUALITY CARING IN ACTION: CLINICAL PRACTICE, EDUCATION, AND LEADERSHIP

Many have envisioned nursing's future, and others have suggested positive, indifferent, or unpleasant scenarios for the future of health care (Bezold, 2005; Trossman, 2002). While some of these stories seem a bit "out there," just a mere 30–40 years ago patients with acute myocardial infarction were hospitalized for three weeks and were maintained in a Coronary Care Unit (CCU) on complete bed rest with no stimulants (coffee or tea) for three days; vaginal childbirth required a 7-day hospitalization; and nurses wore white uniforms, shoes, and caps and worked five 8-hour days and every other weekend! A lot has happened in health care and in nursing during these years, so it is not far-fetched to imagine a different nursing in 2060.

In this case, a more mature nursing workforce will dominate—one whose members are true knowledge-workers—that will lead the health care system in delivering services to those in need. These professionals will be salaried employees who are experts in and use caring as the basis of their work. To do this, they simultaneously make use of both inner and outer resources to provide strength and renewal. In other words, they can replenish themselves or are self-caring.

Professional nurses of the future will have led the transformation from the biomedical, task-oriented, shift-focused approach of today to an alert, confident, engaged professional workforce that is true to its nature, *caring*. Not only does this group have caring capacity, but they embody it—in other words, they work in congruence with their knowledge-base and values. Despite the fact that there are not enough of them, these professionals use their time "in relationship" with patients and families, other health team members, and themselves to promote feeling cared for. They focus on the person rather than the disease and have an appreciation for the larger system in which they work. They are responsible yet flexible, see possibilities, and strive for self-improvement by accepting feedback and continuously learning. Such maturity is not related to age but to a willingness to take the essence of nursing along with current knowledge and recreate a practice that is meaningful, a basis for pride, and that positively impacts patient outcomes (Watson, 1979, 1985). (See Table 10.1 for the Shifting Foci of Professional Nursing.)

In a focus group of recently discharged patients, the following exemplars describe the experience of being "cared for" by mature professional nurses:

A young mother who was separated from her baby due to severe preeclampsia with a resultant admission to the intensive care unit relayed her thoughts about the nurses. "They tailored things to my needs; looked in my eyes; listened and heard; helped me relax so my only job was to get better; *they felt what I felt.*"

A well-educated, 60-year-old woman who was admitted the second time for severe abdominal complications after surgery at another

Table 10.1

THE SHIFTING FOCI OF PROFESSIONAL NURSING

TODAY	2060
Focus on disease	Focus on a person with a disease or health problem
Focus on tasks	Focus on relationships
Adherence to biomedical model	Nursing practice based on nursing models
Focus on a few specialties	All nursing is embraced as special
Focus on a unit as part of an organization	Expanded focus to the system and the community it serves
Focus on the need for administration to make work life better	Focus on self-caring and self-renewal
Victim focus	Pride; focus on nursing's unique and valued contribution

hospital explained the differences she found in her care at this hospital. "On admission to a hospital, patients have a high degree of fear. They want to know that the outcome/s will be the best they can be. The nurses at this hospital maintained their composure, focused on me, made eye contact, used soft voices. They talked and shared information with physicians and each other making sure that information was consistent. *The sense was that I actually mattered, that I got answers, and I never felt scared.*"

A mother shared her experience with her 14-year-old daughter who had major abdominal surgery. She said, *"My daughter was given every opportunity to manage her own care, including her pain. She got educated about her health, and my other children who were visiting benefited.* The overall experience, although unpleasant, taught her a valuable life lesson—to be in control of her health."

A 55-year-old man suffering from chronic alcohol abuse relayed the following: "The nurses had a nonjudgmental mind-set, treated me with respect, provided me with education, and followed up on me. *A typical good nurse is not enough. It takes an exceptional nurse to bring someone out of addiction.*"

The professional caring delivered to these patients generated relaxation, security, knowledge, and hope for recovery; so much so that the patients returned to the hospital to tell their story. The patients were deeply affected by the nurses and believed their recovery was hastened because of them. The nurses expertly practiced the caring factors by placing the patients first; integrating *being* with *doing;* and maintaining a purposeful, inclusive manner; in so doing, they met the needs of their patients.

On the other hand, a young nurse relays the benefits she has gained as a result of her experiences in nursing: "I have grown exponentially as both a person and a nurse . . . My patients helped open my eyes to the diversity of the human experience—different places, situations, and experiences . . . The work is arduous, but the payoffs are some of the best that I have ever experienced: knowing I've used good judgment, admitting when I've made a mistake, applying clinical skills and assessments, knowing I have made an otherwise unbearable situation more pleasant for someone, providing support to those in need, advocating for a patient, helping a coworker, learning to accept help from others, resolving conflict, finding creative solutions, feeling that I am genuinely appreciated" (D'Antonio, 2008, p. 35).

After only two years as a professional, this nurse describes the positive influence her chosen profession has had on her as a human being. Developing and using her caring capacity, she has effectively used her time with patients and families to care, to learn, and to make meaning of her career. In so doing, the nurse has gained many life lessons that have affected her desire for future interactions with patients and families and the continuation of her career. As a matter of fact, Fawcett (2007) takes the stance that practicing true nursing (using nursing's unique theory-driven knowledge) may, in fact, be tied to more available time with patients and families and fewer nursing shortages.

Professional nurses of the future will hold at least a baccalaureate degree, but most will have a graduate degree. As one of several health professionals, professional nurses will forge collaborative relationships with other health team members for the benefit of patients and families and will actively incorporate evidence from quality improvement and research activities into their practice. Robotics and more technological advances will be present but will be considered tools to advance patient care, not the basis for care. The clinical nurse of the future will be admired as an essential member of the health care workforce and will be included in important health care decisions.

Recently, a woman relayed her experience with her husband's nurse as he was preparing for lung surgery. A hospital-based nurse called the patient a week in advance of the surgery at his home to review the upcoming procedure. She spoke about the early postoperative nature of the intensive care unit, the necessary chest tubes, and the pain involved. She coached him on using the 1 to 10 pain scale so they could ensure his comfort. She explained the anticipated length of stay and the recovery period after. While nurses have been doing pre-op teaching for years, thanks to the evidence provided by Lindeman and Van Aernam's (1971) landmark study of the benefits of such teaching, pre-op teaching has become routine. This experience was beneficial to the patient and his wife, but consider how it might unfold in 2060.

A professional nurse working in a hospital perioperative services department introduces himself to the patient and his/her family via a signal transmitted through a pair of eyeglasses. In the comfort of their home, the patient and family see the nurse who initiates a caring relationship with them by using the caring factors during the interaction. The nurse completes an assessment by taking a history and "virtual physical."

During this assessment, the nurse perceives the situation (appreciating what is significant) and then probes, through asking the "right" questions, to classify the data. He/she then synthesizes the data gathered and identifies/prioritizes patient problems. Potential interventions are framed according to the caring factors. In this case, the nurse talks the patient and family through the procedure while they actually "see" it performed through the eyeglasses. The interactions are mutual and questions are encouraged; the nurse uses current literature to provide facts and responds to the family's perceptions based on their own search of the literature. The nurse explains similar procedures he has been involved in and listens intently to the patient and family's individualized way of learning. He administers pre-op functional status and quality of life measures and informs the patient that these will be used again to track his progress and assess the success of the surgery. He is optimistic and offers his contact information. The following week, the family arrives at the hospital one hour before surgery, and the same nurse greets them, completing the pre-op requirements and assuring the patient that he will stay with him during the procedure. He offers the family resources during the wait and then works collaboratively with the entire operating room team to successfully complete the procedure. By the way, the "procedure" may not be in the form of surgery we know today; in fact, a small nanoknife may actually cut away the tumor. The nurse follows the patient to the recovery area (which may not be in ICU) and ensures that the handoff flows smoothly. He stays until the patient is oriented and comfortable and then informs him how the procedure went. The following day, as the patient is getting ready to go home, this nurse reinforces the teaching provided a week earlier, offers guidance to the family, encourages questions and concerns, and sets a time to "meet" the following day. At this meeting, again using a remote system, the nurse checks the patient's vital signs, intake and output, and other physical parameters; ensures his coughing and deep breathing exercises every two hours; and continues to provide information and deal with questions. In addition, he responds to any problems including poor sleeping and low mood or bad feelings, and he offers encouragement. He assesses the need for and timing of his next "visit." Problems arise with this patient in terms of willingness to cough and deep breathe at regular intervals, and a small pneumonia developed. However, the nurse, through increased "visits," detected it early, adjusted the pain medication schedule in collaboration with nurse practitioner colleagues, and provided more coaching. In fact, he actually did the coughing and deep breathing with the patient several times to model how it is best performed! At the end of the first week, the nurse administers the same instruments used pre-op with an additional instrument that measures the *experience of caring* the patient perceived during his surgery. The nurse then enters the data from his own home into the protected perioperative database for analysis. He stays in contact with the patient and family for the next six weeks and then again at an annual follow-up "visit." Additional data are collected on the same instruments at six weeks and one year. The nurse participates in the monthly interprofessional quality improvement meeting where aggregated outcomes data are presented. He contributes to the discussion of increasing morbidity rates after lung surgery by relaying this patient's experience with a setback of pneumonia. The group uses this information, generated from practice, to develop a potential research question, and the nurse agrees to work with his peers on the literature review. In addition, he analyzes the caring factor scores and looks for areas needing improvement. He returns to his family of four each day tired but glad he chose nursing as a profession. During his evening run before dinner, he reflects on his own practice and wonders if he can go to a conference this year on adherence after surgery. And, as a volunteer fireman in his community, he uses his knowledge of nursing to help the community with emergency preparedness. Although the nurse's focus in this example remained on the relationship with the patient and family as well as the health care team, advanced technology was imbedded throughout. He was assigned to several patients at once, although only one example was provided. He demonstrated an ethic of caring that is consistent with the profession combined with an interest and participation in generating evidence for future health care interactions. As Swanson (2008) stated, he was "being a nurse" versus "doing nursing." Receiving outcomes data provided this nurse with feedback on his performance, but more importantly, it highlighted his contribution to the overall health and quality of life of the patients he cared for.

Obviously, a workforce of professional nurses such as the one described requires an educational program that prepares them for this role.

> *Values-based learning* assists students to address the conflicts or tensions between theory and practice and facilitates a greater alignment between the two. In this form of teaching, there are no single best answers but rather differences of opinion that must be explored. Using case examples and real experiences enhances understanding.

Framing the learning experience in a format similar to ethical decision making where facts are exposed, perspectives are clarified, appropriate values are named, alternatives are examined, and eventual decisions are made leads to values-based choices; in this case, caring choices. For example, the following case may be presented to prelicensure students:

> You are a nurse on a busy pediatric unit. One of your patients is a 6-month-old boy who was admitted at 8 lbs, 2 oz. with a "feeding problem" diagnosis. This is his third hospital admission. The young mother states that the boy cries a lot; yet he smiles and has eaten well in your care. You observe the reaction of the child to the mother's significant other (he grimaces and does not seem to want to be held by him). When approaching the pediatrician about your concerns, he tells you that he called protective services in the past about this child. They did a thorough investigation and found no evidence of abuse. So, he proceeded to discharge the child to the mother's care. You feel uneasy and approach your supervisor who agrees with the physician.

Facilitating a class discussion about this case, the faculty member would guide the students to gather facts, name appropriate values that could guide decisions, and choose a course of action. Students would be allowed to disagree and challenge each other resulting in a lively dialogue that would stimulate learning. Or, the following case might be used for senior nursing students who are studying ethics:

> A nurse manager called an emergency staff meeting and announced that she just received a message from the computing center that a patient's medical record had been accessed by persons who were not assigned to the patient. The patient was the wife of the former mayor and had been admitted for "abdominal pain." The nurse manager asked for an explanation, and the group remained silent. One nurse knew what had occurred but declined to relay it in public. After the meeting, she approached the nurse manager and told her about three nurses who thought it would be fun to find out "why the patient was really here." The three nurses were disciplined and accused the reporting nurse of being a rat; they have since stopped talking to her and don't include her in unit activities.

The faculty member would facilitate a conversation about the case using a values-based framework, allowing the students to come to a conclusion about the action of the reporting nurse. At the graduate level, students in an administration program might be presented with the following:

Stan, a 56-year-old night nurse, has worked at a hospital for 24 years. He is a loyal employee and fills in frequently for employees who call in sick. He is well-liked and personable. However, his nurse manager has recently discovered that he is taking food and supplies from the unit and has confronted him. He cites his young daughter who has had recent surgery and needs frequent dressing changes that are taxing his budget. Hospital policy requires termination, but he offers to pay the hospital back and insists he won't do it again.

Using a values-based decision framework, the faculty member would facilitate students to reach a decision for or against termination of the nurse. Using the caring factors, the faculty member gently engages the students, appreciates their input, and suggests possible alternatives. No one definitive answer but multiple opinions may emerge. In both instances, the faculty member helps the students see a course of action that aligns best with caring and produces the greatest benefit to patients and families. Values-based teaching and learning require a comfort with open dialogue and student-led discussions.

Because future nurses will likely be educated at the baccalaureate level, examining these programs in relation to the knowledge required to work in this manner is paramount.

Using a caring approach of shared study, educators will need to value caring relationships as essential to health and be committed to the development of caring knowledge in themselves and their students. To promote a growing awareness of self, students need to be exposed to nursing early in their freshman year and build on the experiences and characteristics they brought to the program. A focus on personal knowing or balancing inner and external knowledge is paramount.

Educational experiences that are open, with mutual dialogue and reflective analysis, enhance such learning. Planned content delivered in lecture format with set course scheduling may not always be the best way to learn and be caring. Caring experiences with patients and families during praxis help students appreciate its value to health care outcomes and their own growth as a caring person. Designing such experiences is a role of the faculty. Crucial to such experiences is asking questions during praxis that stimulate students to think about their experiences with patients and families. Questions such as: What relationships are emerging? What is the quality of the relationships? What seems important to the relationships? and What are the potential consequences of the observed relationships? provide opportunities for much more introspection. Helping students learn the caring factors through study, simulations, and modeling creates situations where students can test their interactions in a safe place under the guidance of experts. Grounding nursing simulations in caring allows faculty to create an environment where the uniqueness of the human person and the fullness of nursing practice can be understood (Eggenberger & Keller, 2008). Likewise, in the online course environment, faculty members must ensure the wholeness of patients and families is preserved. Integrating knowledge from multiple sources is a skill necessary for quality care, so performing this activity early and repeatedly is wise. Finally, ensuring caring competency through formative and summative evaluation helps prepare professional nurses "to be" as well as "to do" nursing.

Interestingly, according to Barry and Purnell (2008), graduate students (who are functioning at rapid paces) often come to educational programs seeking another way of being. They state that "the pedagogical challenge for faculty is to provide an opening for students to slow down, to search inside and to find meaning in their nursing" (p. 19).

At the graduate level, in addition to learning new specialty biomedical content, more time would be better spent looking inward and sharing nursing experiences through reflection and integration among faculty, preceptors, and students. The students' challenge is to find new ways of being that affirms the values of nursing through interpretive activities such as reflective analysis that assist in the development of alternative perspectives and approaches.

Facilitating caring science at the doctoral level through advanced inquiry requires faculty mentors who understand its nature and who are involved with the science themselves. Research mentoring is crucial to build a future group of caring scientists, as is leadership mentoring to build a future group of nursing leaders.

Nurse executives leading upcoming health care institutions will be challenged to *create caring-healing-protective environments for staff and patients that are cost-effective.* Concurrently balancing organizational costs with the human caring needs of patients and staff requires relationship-centered approaches that depend on caring expertise. According to Pappas (2008), the high cost of nursing-sensitive adverse events (those poor outcomes that reflect nursing care) provides information and some justification for specific RN staffing patterns. In this study of 3,230 medical and surgical patients from 2 hospitals in the western United States, "for each additional adverse event, the cost per case increased by $1,020.00" for medical patients and "$903.00" for surgical patients (p. 234). The most frequent nursing-sensitive adverse event found was urinary tract infection (UTI) in both groups of patients, UTI and pressure ulcers in the medical patients, and UTI and pneumonia in the surgical patients. Interestingly, this study adjusted the adverse outcomes for patient age and severity and found that these variables also influenced whether adverse events occurred. Although limited, this study is important because it demonstrates the cost implications of nursing-related adverse outcomes and begins to portray nursing not only as an expense but as a crucial asset to the success of an organization. It also begins to confirm factors that must be taken into consideration for effective and efficient staffing. For example, increased nursing time to assume care for patients without urinary catheters or to facilitate good postoperative pulmonary assessment and airway clearance is crucial to the prevention of nursing-sensitive adverse outcomes. Also, because the older, more severely ill person is more likely to acquire an adverse outcome, these factors must enter into staffing plans. Professional nurses with some added time and competent skills are in a unique position to detect triggers of harm, prevent errors, and ensure safe practice (Institute for Healthcare Improvement, 2006).

Leaders are already being challenged to balance human caring with the economic complexities of the current system. Examining the weekly calendars of most nursing leaders will likely find time spent in multiple meetings, resolving conflicts, or balancing the budget. Little time is left to inspire staff, visit with patients and families (the customer), cultivate meaningful caring relationships with health care colleagues, teach and learn how to improve nursing, or build a lasting legacy for the next generation of nurses. Yet, the value of nursing lies in its caring core. As Swanson and Wojnar (2004) reported, "a caring, healing, integrative approach to health care embraces the importance of sustaining the wholeness of the one caring" (p. S-43). The future will demand leaders who can demonstrate a return on investment for the caring behaviors of professional nurses. Evidence such as increased safety (for both patients and the health care workforce); increased patient satisfaction; faster and better attainment of clinical outcomes; longer-term outcomes such as quality of life, functional status, and return to work; nurse retention; and workforce health will be needed to show how professional nursing influences the performance of a health care system.

Difficult decisions will need to be made *in the best interest of patients and families* in the next few years that will tax nursing leadership (see Table 10.2). For example, research is beginning to show some negative consequences of 12-hour shift scheduling (Rogers, Hwang, Scott, Aiken, & Dinges, 2004; Scott, Rogers, Hwang, & Zhang, 2006). Although originally intended to offer nurses more flexibility and work–life balance while meeting the economic constraints of the health care system (Lorenz, 2008), nurses today either can't seem to leave on time, "volunteer" for more hours and extra shifts, or actually assume another job on their time off. This has resulted in a tired workforce, poor continuity of patient care, and, in some cases, medical errors. The question for nursing administration is whether 12-hour scheduling is beneficial to patients and families and the nurses themselves. Lorenz (2008) poses this question as an ethical one because the interests of patients and families are cited as the *first priority* of health care executives (American College of Health Care Executives, 2007). Another recent study of nurse scheduling examined the mix of shifts nurses work (e.g., 4-hour, 6-hour, 8-hour, and 12-hour) to see whether this chaotic pattern with resultant multiple handoffs contributed to patient safety and quality (Kalisch, Begeny, & Anderson, 2008). The results showed an influence on teamwork and continuity of care, and implications for decreasing the number of different shifts were suggested. In a time of nursing shortage where staff nurses want flexible scheduling, nursing leaders are faced with this preliminary evidence that requires thoughtful decision making.

Redesigning clinical work, including rethinking the nature of tasks and relationships, is a national priority. Consider how acute care nurses use their time during a shift. First, they spend about one hour receiving reports from the prior shift—oftentimes this is not comprehensive or relationship-enhancing. Next, they organize themselves according to the various tasks—assessments, medication administration, and treatments that need completion. Then, as they proceed down the list of tasks, they

Table 10.2

LEADERSHIP DECISIONS NECESSARY FOR THE FUTURE OF NURSING

1. Balance caring-healing-protective environments for staff and patients with costs

2. Safe staffing—assure the appropriate number of professional nurses for individual patients' human caring needs

3. Appraise nurse scheduling to respect flexibility while ensuring continuity of services and decreased opportunities for human error

4. Redesign clinical work that integrates *being* and *doing* caring

5. Address workplace abuse and violence

6. Empower nursing leadership at all levels to express caring

are checked off one by one until finally documentation, which is typically saved until last, appears. At this point, they save up all this information and report it to the oncoming nurse. One or two disruptions or emergencies can throw the entire checklist off, necessitating overtime in order to complete the list. But, during this 8–12-hour period, one of the patients received a cancer diagnosis, another did not achieve pain relief, another patient requiring a complex dressing change after discharge was told by his daughter that she would not be able to take him home with her, and a physician on the staff just found out his daughter was admitted to the psych ward for bulimia. In the busyness of completing the checklist, how aware were the nurses on this unit of the complexities of their patients' or coworkers' lives? Or for that matter, their own stomachs or bladders?

Patients and families desire information, reassurance, acceptance, support, commitment, kindness, acknowledgment, competence, mutual decision making, vigilance, comfort, security, family engagement, and their basic human needs met (Duffy et al., 2007; Fomella & Sheldon, 2004). They want to be treated as if they were a close relative of the care provider; they want to matter. And don't we all? Nurses consistently say they want to relate to their patients and work with other nurses who perform the same way (Studer Group, 2005). In other words, they want a caring-healing-protective environment. Yet, all predictions point to a lower supply of professional nurses. Designing care delivery models that incorporate caring relationships with fewer RNs requires careful, reflective analysis of the work of professional nursing, identification of the role dimensions of future professional nurses, and tough decisions about how that work will be accomplished. Included in this analysis must be the fundamental understanding that nursing incorporates *both being* with and *doing* for in an integrated fashion. This is known as clinical integrity.

It is in the daily, oftentimes ordinary, processes of feeding, bathing, changing dressings, administering medications, or ambulating that nurses relate to patients in an intimate manner at some of the most vulnerable times of life. Completing these tasks affords the opportunity to accurately understand from the patient's point of view what is important and design individualized patient-sensitive interventions.

Expert nurses incorporate the caring factors during these activities, and in so doing, they create health experiences that are safe, comfortable, optimistic, and that preserve the wholeness of persons. In other words, competent nurse work consists of specific actions delivered in a particular patient-defined context. A well-represented national think-tank or study of the future role of professional nursing may be a preliminary step toward better understanding of professional nurse work. The roles of front-line managers and other health care leaders will be modified to accommodate such care delivery models. Dramatic restructuring of nursing work with resulting implications for staffing, scheduling, and the work of other health professionals will follow.

Affectively addressing abuse and violence in the workplace is another arduous but necessary leadership responsibility. Caring relationships minimally demand civil discourse; expecting caring relationships at all levels requires relationship-centered leadership with skills in consensus building, conflict resolution, and maintaining a work focus on the patient and family. Understanding how abusive nurses impact the rest of the health care team and dealing effectively with them, including letting them go if necessary, is imperative. In fact, the Joint Commission on Accreditation of Healthcare (JCAHO) has recently called attention to and created standards dealing with disruptive and inappropriate workplace behaviors (JCAHO, 2008). These standards specifically hold leaders accountable for consistently ensuring acceptable professional behavior. Without such leadership, good nurses may eventually leave or, worse, resign themselves to the situation and stagnate. This is not in the best interest of quality patient care.

Maintaining a team of first-line managers who focus primarily on caring relationships is another leadership challenge. Today's performance expectations of first-line managers have positioned them uncomfortably between staff and administration. On the one hand, they are responsible for quality patient care, and on the other hand, they are asked to prepare reports, attend meetings, attain another degree, or reconcile the budget. The real work of first-line nurse managers of the future will be to create safe, open, flexible environments that successfully safeguard patients and families, preserve the integrity of professional nursing, and contain organizational costs. This requires global awareness; analytical and sophisticated research and evaluation capacity; expert interpersonal relationship skills; self-caring ability; advanced knowledge of nursing, including nursing theory and professional practice models; the ability to collaborate, share successes, and acknowledge failures; and most importantly, the ability to express caring. Just as with staff nurses and educators, a shortage of first-line and executive-level nursing leadership is predicted (Sherman & Bishop, 2007). Now is the time to shore up first-line nurse managers to build teams capable of renewing nursing. Some nurse executives have already started this by creating self-caring teams of nurse managers. One example includes a medical–surgical division in an acute care hospital with eight nurse managers who regularly meet weekly for one hour just to "check in," participate in a book club (of relevant readings), and attend off-campus gatherings once a month to work on mutual goals and support each other; they are only allowed to bring or order "healthy" foods during these group meetings. In addition, the vice president for patient care services at this organization partners with the local nursing program in an annual nursing renewal ceremony. The students have an annual commitment ceremony at this school that replaces the more traditional capping ceremony. The hospital in partnership with the nursing program has begun participating by sending its nursing staff and leadership and often furnishing the guest speaker. During the ceremony the entire group (students and nurses alike) recites the International Pledge for Professional Nursing. This ceremony usually takes place in the fall and helps to honor and renew professional nursing. First-line managers in this organization know that their primary role is to "be" caring.

In a 2008 review summary regarding sustaining nursing leadership that fosters a healthy work environment; collaboration; increased education; the ability to motivate, communicate, support, listen, and manage conflict; and ongoing professional development were synthesized from 48 qualitative studies as necessary leadership qualities (The Joanna Briggs Institute, 2008). Expecting and ensuring that future front-line nurse managers have the knowledge and skills necessary to keep the focus on caring relationships means making hard decisions about who will be hired, how persons will be evaluated and rewarded, who will be retained, and how persons will be prepared. The future will demand a *minimum* masters preparation for the first-line manager and a doctoral preparation for executive leadership.

According to Roy (2000), the principles upon which nursing administrators should plan for the future include unity, maximizing human potential, and promise. Unity suggests less boundaries and more harmony, partnership, collaboration, and integration. Maximizing human potential first recognizes the word *human*—multidimensional beings—and *potential,* or possibilities. Maximizing human potential realizes that humans are capable of advancing and through relationships can grow and change. Promise indicates hope. Each of these principles hinges on relationships. Nursing leaders who embrace caring relationships will step up to the plate and make the hard decisions required for radical and lasting professional renewal.

NURSING'S PROMISING FUTURE

Cornish (2004) affirmed that history teaches us how to approach new frontiers by learning from the explorers of every age. In his text *Futuring: The Exploration of the Future,* he recounted the lessons of earlier explorers (pp. 1–8). They are:

Prepare carefully

Anticipate needs

Use available information

Expect the unexpected

Think long- AND short-term

Dream productively

Learn from your predecessors

Using these principles as a guide, nursing has a real opportunity to provide evidence of its value, improve patient care, generate new ways of doing nurse work, and advance the profession. Preparing for a system of complexity means sitting down and planning how to cope or rather transcend the difficulties presented to us. Anticipating by identifying potential needs and imagining how to meet them using available practical guidance helps one make decisions in situations that require immediate action. Expecting unforeseen circumstances helps garner the resources required to master them before they occur. Long-term thinking, while simultaneously managing the present, allows goals to become reality. And *productive* dreaming sustains the long-term thinking, enabling the achievement of realistic goals, including the strategies for getting there. Finally, placing a heavy emphasis on lessons learned from the past helps prevent mistakes. Taken together, these principles have guided the evolution of the Quality-Caring Model such that it incorporates a longer-term, more holistic, integrated set of relationships from which to guide professional practice.

We are beginning to appreciate the significance of caring relationships as the basis for professional nursing. Acknowledging this uniqueness and demonstrating a professional commitment to it offer a way for nursing to survive as a flourishing profession. It is in the ordinary everyday actions of professional nurses that transforming experiences occur. These experiences occur in *both* patients and nurses and provide opportunities of real meaning—witnessing a couple in love with their newborn baby, eye contact with another nurse while turning a bed-bound patient, understanding seen in the eyes of a male ventilator-dependent patient after an explanation about his constant secretions, sitting with a family gathered by the bedside of a dying person, the slight smile on a young boy's face who finally had enough courage to give himself an insulin injection after learning from a nurse, the appreciation of an employee for counseling provided—all create possibilities. Embodying caring—giving it form—demonstrating who we are as human beings; living and working in a way that integrates body, mind, soul; and creating community partnerships lead to a wholeness or synthesis that influences future interactions and advancement.

According to Swanson (2008), the outcomes influenced by nurses who practice this way include: helping patients and families feel understood, valued, safe, comfortable, capable/confident, and hopeful. These outcomes are a compelling witness to professional nursing! In another dimension, however, individual nurses themselves can benefit from caring professional practice. Although illness can be sad, it also creates the possibility for patients and families to pause from life's busyness and do some introspection as they try to make sense of their illness. Patients who are sick tend to be doing just that as they lie in wait for diagnostic tests or recovery; nurses can access those life lessons everyday through caring relationships!

Turmoil and instability sometimes prevent consideration of what really matters—in this case, professional nursing's primary function, caring relationships. But, it is precisely at this time that pondering the essence of nursing may provide the strength necessary to carry out dramatic change. Professional nurses are educated primarily to care but programmed by the work environment to carry out multiple tasks as if they were independent from caring relationships. This creates tension and discord and leads to job dissatisfaction. Uniting the caring core of nursing with the scientific principles of inquiry will provide nursing with theory-guided, evidence-based professional practice that is holistic and meaningful (Watson, 1979, 1985). Kitson (1996) reminds us that nursing's roots were born in a period of social reform, scientific advancement, and controversy. Blending nursing's fundamental nature, *caring*, with the continued search for excellence will enable the profession to advance and thrive. One hospital participated in a future search visioning exercise over several months. Through the process that involved all levels of nursing, they forged new relationships built on trust and a leveling of hierarchy, and they discovered common ground about nursing that was filled with hope, enthusiasm, and wonder for the future (Capuano, Durichin, Millard, & Hitchings, 2007). This nursing group got engaged and created the future of nursing in their organization.

Taking advantage of this time in history to make a profound impact on patient outcomes will revitalize professional nursing. Some would argue that professional nursing will be determined by those outside the profession. Others believe it is a moral imperative of nursing to leave a legacy of caring and quality (Johnstone & Kanitsaki, 2006; Watson, 2006). Whatever one's stance on the future of nursing, vulnerable, dependent, sometimes poor, and often fearful patients *need* to feel secure about the intentions, actions, and professional competence of nurses. The profession's future rests on all of us.

SUMMARY

Reflections about the future were presented. Particular attention was paid to health care, including projected technological advances, continued cost pressure, and the challenges of a growing complex system. A sophisticated nursing workforce will be needed that understands the "big picture" and practices from a caring stance. The revised Quality-Caring Model provides a framework for such practice and offers persons with health needs experiences that preserve their wholeness and advance self-caring. Assumptions and propositions of the model are included, and the role of the nurse is specified. Nursing in 2060 is envisioned with examples, and a values-based learning approach is described as one method of preparing future nurses. Multiple forms of nursing education (e.g., classroom, simulation, online) that are grounded in caring as well as the development of synthesis skills were emphasized. Making difficult decisions in the best interest of patients and families such as staffing, scheduling, addressing workplace violence, and maintaining caring-focused front-line nurse managers were stressed as important to future nursing leaders. Rethinking the work of nursing in order to effect lasting change for professional nursing was considered a major leadership charge for the immediate future. Finally, embracing caring relationships as the basis for practice offers professional nursing a promising future that will make a profound impact on patient outcomes.

CALLS TO ACTION

Relationships, specifically caring relationships, as the basis for actions and decision-making are necessary to discover the clinical and organizational knowledge that already exists in health care systems. Highly developed, inclusive, and interdependent professional nurses who understand the significance of the whole and whose practice is based on caring evidence are needed to generate the critical mass needed for lasting change. **Identify** the caring leaders you can turn to for guidance.

Using the knowledge of caring relationships as the basis for its work, nursing validates the nature of humans as they exist in union with the universe. **Consider** how nursing serves society.

(continued)

The caring factors ground human relationships such that a connection occurs that is transpersonal (more than the individuals alone). Transpersonal relationships lead to knowing the other; knowing another facilitates actions such as anticipation, guidance, providing for, teaching and learning, protecting, and advocating. Human relationships that are transpersonal create possibilities for development and progress in all those involved. **Experiment** with ways to deepen your knowledge of "the other."

The dynamic, progressive nature of excellent health care systems reflects the caring ability of its workforce. Employees who cultivate caring relationships with themselves, their communities, patients and families, and among members of the health care team contribute to an organization's health. That is, an organization's capacity to find its strengths, change, learn, and adapt, particularly during difficult times, is dependent on the caring relationships of its employees. **Discover and imitate** the caring experts in your organization.

A mindful, engaged, and scientific professional workforce that remains true to its caring roots will help shift the biomedical, task-oriented, shift-focused approach of today to an interactive, whole-system, theory-based practice that invigorates the health care system. Regularly **participate** in self-awareness practices and research.

Nursing educators who value caring relationships as essential to health will further the development of caring knowledge. **Internalize** the significance of caring relationships to health.

Rethinking the task-focused work of professional nursing is a national priority. The nonlinear and multiple relationships so common to health care work require a completely different focus of attention—one that embraces little structure and form but allows for relationships to generate ideas and conditions for innovation. The goal of the leader is to enable the health care system to emerge and self-advance by increasing the number and quality of interactions, developing caring-healing-protective environments, and being mindful of the unfolding world in which they function. **Generate** new ways of thinking about nursing work.

(continued)

Demonstrating a return on investment for the caring behaviors of professional nurses will be a leadership responsibility. **Offer** some practical evidence of nursing's value to your organization.

Reflective analysis of the future work of professional nursing, including the identification of role dimensions, will require difficult decisions about how that work will be accomplished. **Think about** the meaning in patient encounters, including the technical skill required.

Expecting caring relationships in all interactions minimally demands civil discourse. Nontolerance for verbal or other abuse in the workplace starts with relationship-centered leadership that continuously focuses on what's best for patients and families. **Role model** caring relationships.

How front-line nurse managers will be prepared, hired, evaluated, rewarded, and retained for a work environment focused on caring relationships will require in-depth analysis and crucial decision making. **Challenge** front-line nurse managers to **embrace** caring professional practice models.

Weaving the caring core of nursing with the scientific principles of inquiry strengthens and forms new connections that will influence the future direction of professional nursing. **Engender** hope and possibility.

Reflective Questions/Applications for Students

1. Discuss professional nursing practice in 2060. What will the work environment look like? What actions will make up the majority of nursing time?
2. In preparing for tomorrow's professional nurse, what do you consider are the top five needs? What can we glean from the pioneers in nursing that may help this transition?
3. What do we need to do as a profession to better prepare nurses of the future for the challenges that await them?

4. What attitudes need to change?
5. What do we want to conserve about nursing?
6. Discuss the philosophical and theoretical underpinnings of the Quality-Caring Model. How do Donabedian (1966), Watson (1979), King (1981), and Irvine et al. (1998) inform the model?
7. Explain how the caring factors assist in protecting patients from harm. Be specific.
8. List and discuss five assumptions of the Quality-Caring Model.
9. Discuss the pros and cons of salaried professional nurses.
10. Create a future scenario (25 years from now) of a patient situation from your area of expertise. What is different about professional nursing, and what remains the same?

Reflective Questions/Applications for Educators

11. Describe how a values-based approach to a sophomore nursing course could be initiated. What would be required of faculty? Students? How would the course be evaluated?
12. What are the necessary thinking patterns that will have to occur in graduate students in order to meet the challenges of relationship-centered caring?
13. Create a future clinical nursing scenario either for the simulation lab or for use as a case study. Evaluate it with real students and revise as necessary.
14. Design a leadership course introducing the Quality-Caring Model. Include objectives and an evaluation mechanism. How would you know if the students could apply the model to their practice?
15. Choose a proposition from the revised Quality-Caring Model. Using a population of interest, present a research question that could test this proposition. Include relevant variables and hypotheses. What instruments might be used to test your hypotheses?
16. Evaluate the necessity of introducing nursing courses early (first semester) in a baccalaureate academic program?
17. Discuss with fellow faculty members the redesign and testing of one undergraduate and one graduate course using a values-based approach. What would the objectives look like? Who would teach it? How would the students and faculty be evaluated?

Reflective Questions/Applications for Nurse Leaders

18. Record the methodology you would use to justify increased RN staffing for a nursing unit with the majority population older than 65 years.

19. Examine Table 10.2. Provide some input/suggestions into the resolution of these difficult decisions keeping in mind the "best interest of patients and families."

20. Create a plan for dramatically altering RN work at your organization. Who would be involved? What methodology would be used? How long would it take? What implications for RN staffing and scheduling would occur? How would you ensure that all opinions and ideas were heard?

21. What critical knowledge and skills concerning caring relationships has the nursing leadership team in your organization acquired? What caring knowledge and skills do they lack? Create a plan for attaining the requisite knowledge and skills for relationship-centered caring.

22. How do *you* help nurses stay focused on caring relationships in their day-to-day practice?

23. What can nurse leaders do to ensure that professional nurses will focus on the "big picture" and be willing to accept the challenges of self-caring?

24. What will your legacy be? What will you leave the next generation of nurses and patients?

25. How does *quality* currently fit within your everyday practice?

REFERENCES

American College of Health Care Executives. (2007). *ACHE Code of Ethics.* Retrieved May 7, 2008, from http://www.ache.org/ABT_ACHE/code.cfm

Antrobus, S. (1997). Developing the nurse as a knowledge worker in health-learning: The artistry of practice. *Journal of Advanced Nursing, 25*(4), 829–835.

Barry, C., & Purnell, M. J. (2008). Uncovering meaning through the aesthetic turn: A pedagogy of caring. *International Journal for Human Caring, 12*(2), 19–23.

Batalden, P. B., & Davidoff, F. (2007). What is "quality improvement" and how can it transform healthcare? *Quality and Safe Health Care, 16*, 2–3.

Benford, G., & Malartre, E. (2007). *Beyond human: Living with robots and cyborgs.* New York: Tom Doherty Associates, LLC.

Berwick, D. M. (2008). The science of improvement. *Journal of the American Medical Association, 299*(10), 1182–1184.

Bezold, C. (2005). The future of patient-centered care: Scenarios, visions, and audacious goals. *Journal of Alternative and Complementary Medicine, 11*(Suppl. 1), s-77–s-84.

Butler, R. N. (2008). *The longevity revolution: The benefits and challenges of living a long life.* New York: Perseus Book Group.

Canton, J. (2006). *The extreme future: The top ten trends that will reshape the world for the next 5, 10, and 20 years.* New York: Penguin Group.

Capuano, T., Durichin, L. D., Millard, J. L., & Hitchings, K. S. (2007). The desired future of nursing doesn't just happen—engaged nurses create it. *Journal of Nursing Administration, 37*(2), 61–63.

Chopra, D. (2008). *The third Jesus.* New York: Harmony Books.

Cornish, E. (2004). *Futuring: The exploration of the future.* Bethesda, MD: World Future Society.

D'Antonio, M. (2008). Why I almost quit nursing. *Johns Hopkins Nursing, 6*(2), 34–35.

Donabedian, A. (1966). Evaluating the quality of medical care. *Milbank Memorial Fund Quarterly: Health and Society, 44*(3, Pt. 2), 166–203.

Duffy, J., Hoskins, L. M., & Seifert, R. F. (2007). Dimensions of caring: Psychometric properties of the caring assessment tool. *Advances in Nursing Science, 30*(3), 235–245.

Eggenberger, T. L., & Keller, K. B. (2008). Grounding nursing simulations in caring: An innovative approach. *International Journal for Human Caring, 12*(2), 42–46.

Fawcett, J. (2007). Nursing qua nursing: The connection between nursing knowledge and nursing shortages. *Journal of Advanced Nursing, 59*(1), 97–99.

Fawcett, J., Watson, J., Neuman, B., Hinton-Walker, P., & Fitzpatrick, J. J. (2001). On nursing theories and evidence. *Nursing Administration Quarterly, 33*(2), 115–119.

Fomella, N., & Sheldon, R. (2004). Creating a desirable future for nursing, Part 2: The issues. *Journal of Nursing Administration, 34*(6), 264–267.

Foresight Nanotech Institute. (2008). *Nanotechnology provides two-compartment nanoparticles for drug delivery.* Retrieved September 11, 2008, from http://www.foresight.org/nanodot/?p=2837

Ginsburg, G. S., & McCarthy, J. J. (2001). Personalized medicine: Revolutionizing drug discovery and patient care. *Trends in Biotechnology, 19*(1), 491–496.

Heckel, A. (2008). *More describe selves as spiritual, not religious.* Retrieved May 9, 2008, from http://www.dailycamera.com/news/2008/apr/27/more-describe-selves-as-spiritual-not-religious/

The Henry J. Kaiser Family Foundation. (2007). *Employee health benefits: 2007 annual survey.* Retrieved May 9, 2008, from http://www.kff.org/insurance/7672/index.cfm

Horn, S. D., & Gassaway, J. (2007). Practice-based evidence study design for comparative effectiveness research. *Medical Care, 45*(10, Suppl. 2), S50–S57.

Institute for Healthcare Improvement. (2006). *IHI global trigger tool for measuring adverse events.* Cambridge, MA: Author.

Irvine, D., Sidani, S., & McGillis Hall, L. (1998). Linking outcomes to nurses' roles in health care. *Nursing Economics, 16*(2), 58–64.

The Joanna Briggs Institute. (2008). Comprehensive systematic review of evidence on developing and sustaining nursing leadership that fosters a healthy work environment in health care. *Journal of Advanced Nursing, 62*(6), 653–654.

Johnstone, M. J., & Kanitsake, O. (2006). The moral imperative of designating patient safety and quality care as a national nursing research priority. *Collegian, 13*(1), 5–9.

The Joint Commission on Accreditation of Healthcare Organizations (JCAHO). (2008). Behaviors that undermine a culture of safety. *Sentinel Event Alert, 40*. Retrieved August 22, 2008, from http://www.jointcomission.org/SentinelEvents/SentinelEventAlert/sea_40.htm

Kalisch, B. J., Begeny, S., & Anderson, C. (2008). The effect of consistent nursing shifts on teamwork and continuity of care. *Journal of Nursing Administration, 38*(3), 132–137.

King. I. (1981). *A theory for nursing: Systems, concepts, process.* New York: John Wiley.

Kitson, A. L. (1996). Does nursing have a future? *British Medical Journal, 313*(7072), 1647–1651.

Kondro, W. (2007). American Medical Association boards implantable chip wagon. *Canadian Medical Association Journal, 177*(4), 131–132.

Lanfear, D. E., & McLeod, H. L. (2007). Pharmacogenetics: Using DNA to optimize drug therapy. *American Family Physician, 76*(8), 1179–1182.

Lindemann, C. A., & Van Aerman, B. V. (1971). Nursing intervention with the presurgical patient: The effect structures and unstructural preoperative teaching. *Nursing Research, 20,* 319–332.

Lorenz, S. G. (2008). 12-hour shifts: An ethical dilemma for the nurse executive. *Journal of Nursing Administration, 38*(6), 297–301.

Lusk, B. (1997). Professional classifications of American Nurses, 1910 to 1935. *Western Journal of Nursing Research, 19*(2), 227–242.

National Nanotechnology Initiative (NNI). (2008). *About the NNI.* Retrieved May 13, 2008, from http://www.nano.gov/html/about/home_home-about.html

Neame, R. (1997). Smart cards—The key to trustworthy health information systems. *British Medical Journal, 314,* 573.

Nightingale, F. (1992). *Notes on nursing* (Com. Ed). Philadelphia, PA: Lippincott Publishing.

Pappas, S. H. (2008). The cost of nurse-sensitive adverse events. *Journal of Nursing Administration, 38*(5), 230–236.

Pawson, R., & Tilley, N. (1997). *Realistic evaluation.* London: Sage Publications.

Poisal, J. A., Truffer, C., Smith, S., Sisko, A., Cowan, C., Keehan, S., et al. (2007). Health spending projections through 2016: Modest changes obscure Part D's impact. *Health Affairs, 26*(2), W242–253.

Rogers, A. E., Hwang, W. T., Scott, L. D., Aiken, L. H., & Dinges, D. F. (2004). The working hours of hospital staff nurses and patient safety. *Health Affairs (Millwood), 23,* 202–212.

Roy, C. (2000). A theorist envisions the future and speaks to nursing administrators. *Nursing Administration Quarterly, 24*(2), 1–12.

Scott, L., Rogers, A., Hwang, W., & Zhang, Y. (2006). Effects of critical care nurses; Work hours on vigilance and patients' safety. *American Journal of Critical Care, 15,* 30–37.

Senge, P. (1990). *The fifth discipline: The art and practice of the learning organization.* New York: Doubleday.

Sherman, R. O., & Bishop, M. (2007). The role of nursing educators in grooming future nurse leaders. *Journal of Nursing Education, 46*(7), 295–296.

Sidani, S., & Braden, C. J. (1998). *Evaluating nursing interventions: A theory-driven approach*. Thousand Oaks, CA: Sage Publications.

Studer Group. (2005). *How (and why) to nurture your nurses all year-round*. Retrieved March 21, 2008, from http://www.studergroup.com/dotCMS/knowledgeAssetDetail?inode=238269

Swanson, K. (1991). Empirical development of a middle range theory of caring. *Nursing Research, 40,* 161–166.

Swanson, K. (2008). *Continuing the development of caring theory* (oral presentation). Chapel Hill, NC: 30th Annual International Association for Human Caring Conference.

Swanson, K., & Wojnar, D. M. (2004). Optimal healing environments in nursing. *The Journal of Alternative and Complementary Medicine, 10*(Suppl. 1), s-43–s-48.

Tippett, K. (2008). Speaking of faith: The spirituality of parenting. *American Public Media.* Retrieved March 21, 2008, from http://speakingoffaith.publicradio.org/programs/spiritualityofparenting/yourvoices.shtml

Trossman, S. (2002). Envisioning a brighter future. *American Journal of Nursing, 102*(7), 65–66.

Watson, J. (1979). *Nursing: The philosophy and science of caring*. Boston: Little, Brown and Company.

Watson, J. (1985). *Nursing: Human science and human care*. New York: National League for Nursing.

Watson, J. (2006). Caring theory as ethical guide to administrative and clinical practices. *Journal of Nursing Administration, 8*(1), 87–93.

World Future Society. (2008). *World future 2008*. Retrieved May 9, 2008, from http://www.wfs.org

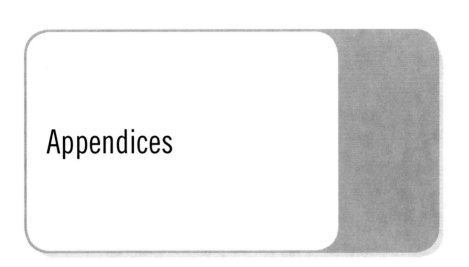

Appendices

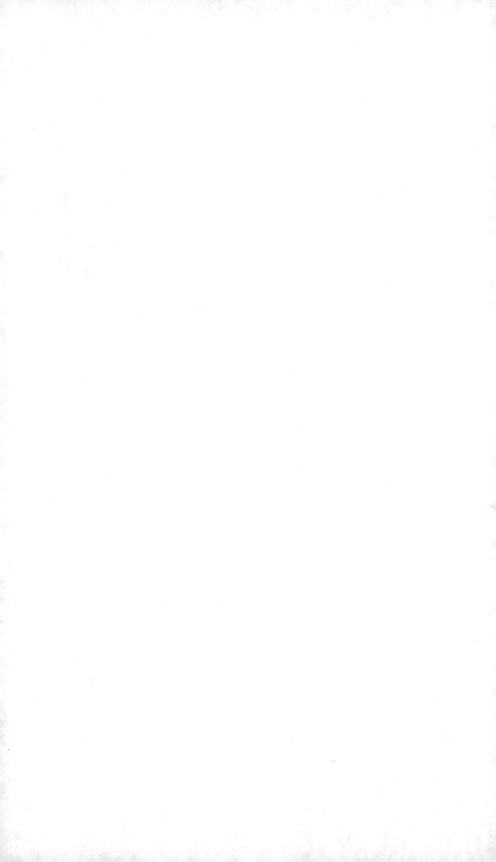

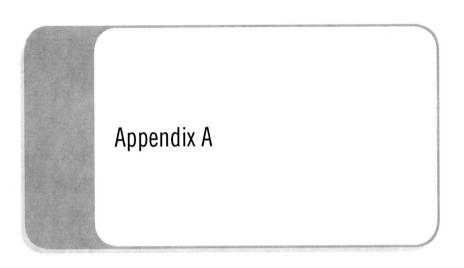

Appendix A

QUALITY- AND CARING-BASED RESOURCES ON THE INTERNET

The Berkana Institute (http://www.berkana.org/)
The Caritas Consortium (http://www.caritasconsortium.org/)
Institute of Noetic Sciences (http://www.noetic.org/)
International Association for Human Caring (http://www.human caring.org)
The National Center for Nursing Quality (http://www.nursing quality.org/)
Nursing Theory Link Page (http://nursing.clayton.edu/eichel berger/nursing.htm)
Nursing Theory Page (http://www.sandiego.edu/ACADEMICS/ nursing/theory/)
The Plexus Institute (http://www.plexusinstitute.org)
Relationship-centered Care Initiative (http://meded.iusm.iu.edu/ resources/rcciinfo.htm)
Society for Organizational Learning (http://www.solonline.org/ aboutsol/)
Watson Caring Science Institute (http://www.watsoncaringscience. org)

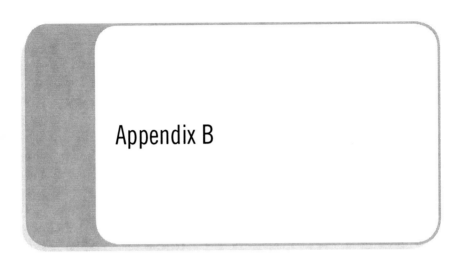

Appendix B

IMPLICATIONS OF THE QUALITY-CARING MODEL©

Common to All Nurses

1. Develop caring capacity for relating to self, patients, and families (or students, staff nurses); health care team members; and the community
2. Learn and practice the caring factors
3. Recognize the value of theory-based practice to professional nursing and quality health outcomes

Nurses in Clinical Practice

4. Advance your education
5. Let nursing theory guide your practice
6. Use your work time wisely—focus on the two relationships necessary for quality
7. Use the caring factors to effectively collaborate with health team members
8. Build in time during the work day to remind yourself why you are there
9. Listen to your patients—they are the best source of information

Nurse Educators

10. Set the tone for student success
11. Increase contact with students
12. Preserve reciprocity between students and faculty
13. Choose values-based teaching–learning strategies
14. Increase clinical learning experiences
15. Test the Quality-Caring Model©
16. Provide prompt feedback to students
17. Develop orientation and continuing education programs to support caring knowledge and skills
18. Mentor emerging caring scientists
19. Use evaluation techniques that are meaningful

Nurse Leaders

20. Use professional practice models as a foundation for nursing practice
21. Revise roles and responsibilities of nurse leaders
22. Partner in demonstration projects
23. Revise career development programs
24. Recognize, reward, and incentivize nurses for their caring practice
25. Make tough decisions in the best interest of patients and families
26. Regularly renew/celebrate the caring spirit of nursing in your organization
27. Care for yourself, your staff, your patients, and your community

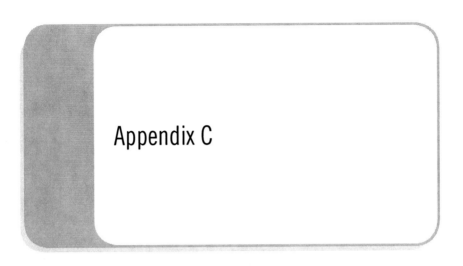

Appendix C

REFLECTIONS FOR CLINICAL PRACTICE

- Think about someone you have experienced as a caring leader and identify some of their key attributes. List them.
- Reflect on an unhappy experience in your career. Write down some concrete examples or strategies that you used that were (a) helpful and (b) not helpful.
- Pretend you are intubated.

  What would you want from your nurse?
  What would you most want to say?
  How would you most likely communicate your needs, especially pain?
  What would be most important to you?

- Remember a time when you really connected with a patient/family. What was going on around you? What inner sense do you recall that might have energized you?
- Call to mind the activities you performed during your last shift. What did you primarily focus on? Did the activities create a sense of feeling "cared for" in your patients? How do you know? How did the time spent at work affect you?

- Think about the last time you asked a patient, "How are you today?" Did you really want to know the answer? What could you have done differently?
- Observe the attachment you might have to the hurried, multitasking nursing environment. How often do you talk about it—with other nurses, at home? What pleasure do you derive from it? Be truthful.
- Consider the wisdom of professional nurses. Where does it come from? How can you more easily tap into it?

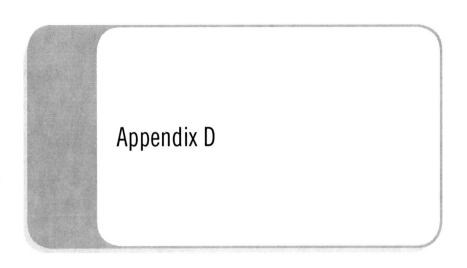

Appendix D

USING THE CARING FACTORS TO KEEP PATIENTS SAFE

Help patients and families understand the threats to their safety.
Listen to their concerns.
Clarify questions.
Routinely check, make rounds offering assistance with basic
   needs.
Anticipate their needs.
Assure availability.
Call patients and families by name.
Allow patients to choose when and where they receive care.
Remove noxious stimuli—lights, noise, and so on.
Position and reposition often.
Know what is important to patients.
Relieve muscle tension through range of motion, massage, exer-
   cises, and relaxation techniques.
Provide fast and effective pain relief.
Assist patients with food, sleeping arrangements, and elimination.
Maintain privacy and confidentiality.
Be alert for variables that are threats to safety.
Provide gentle, sensitive physical care.
Provide anticipatory guidance.

Engage family members in patients' care and decision making.

Communicate (including shift report) at the bedside, including the patient in the discussion.

Use consistent verbal and nonverbal behaviors.

Show patients they can depend on you by walking the talk.

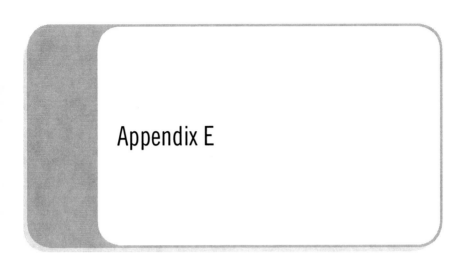

Appendix E

COURSE OBJECTIVES AND CONTENT OUTLINE FOR A STAFF NURSE RESEARCH INTERNSHIP IN HUMAN CARING

Objectives

At the end of this program, students will be able to:

1. Describe the major concepts, assumptions, and propositions of several caring theories.
2. Link caring professional practice to nursing-sensitive patient outcomes.
3. Analyze the components of caring-based nursing interventions.
4. Choose an instrument for the measurement of caring.
5. Apply a research method to the study of caring in nursing.

Content Outline

   I. Overview of human caring theories
  II. Nursing-sensitive patient outcomes
 III. Caring-based nursing interventions

IV. Instruments used to measure caring
V. Research methodologies in caring science

Evaluation

Completion of a mentored research study.

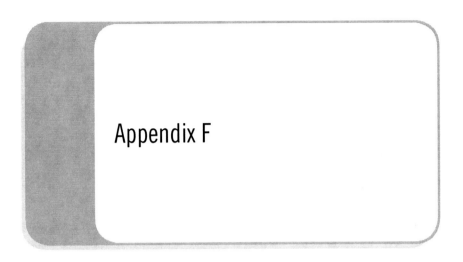

Appendix F

ASSESSMENT OF CARING PROFESSIONAL PRACTICE

Directions: To answer the following question: **Where is caring evidenced at your institution?** evaluate the following structure, process, and outcome variables for the presence and/or linkage to the caring factors. Next, evaluate how well they were represented on a scale from 1 (poor) to 5 (extremely well). (Note: Higher scores [range from 22–110] reflect better representation of caring professional practice.)

Admission Database

Pathways/care plans—are they nurse or patient driven?
Documentation system

Daily processes

Shift report
Rounds/Physician visits
Delegation of responsibilities to patient care assistants
The admission process
Patient education materials
Discharge planning processes
Decision making at unit level

Family visitation
Policy and procedure manual

Physical environment

Family waiting areas
Bulletin boards
Meeting areas and learning resources for staff
Staff meetings
Scheduling/staffing
Assignments

Patient Outcomes

Routinely measured nursing-sensitive outcomes
Shared outcomes measured
Feedback mechanism for outcomes reporting

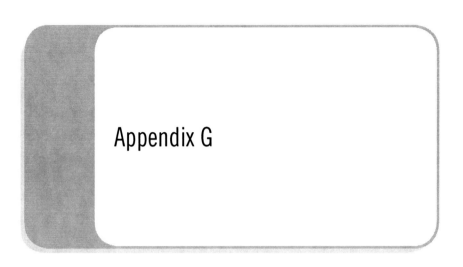

Appendix G

POTENTIAL RESEARCH QUESTIONS FOR CARING SCIENCE

What difference do caring relationships make in specific nursing-sensitive outcomes?

What are the qualities of environments and communities that are considered to be caring?

How does nurse caring influence patient outcomes in multiple settings or patient populations (e.g., long-term care, schools, home health care)?

What structure and process factors influence nurse caring capacity?

How effective are caring-based interventions on health promotion, quality of life, self-caring, decreased symptoms, illness knowledge, and hospital readmission rates?

What is the relationship between nurse caring capacity and patient safety?

What is the cost/benefit of caring professional practice?

What is the relationship between nursing leadership and caring capacity?

What are the psychometric properties of caring tools for specialized populations (e.g., pediatrics)?

How do professional nurses and patients differ in terms of nurse caring capacity?

What improvements in nursing-sensitive patient outcomes are linked to nurse caring?

What is the nature of the student–teacher relationship? In undergraduates? In graduate students?

What is the relationship between faculty caring and student learning?

How does caring practice affect system outcomes (e.g., LOS, costs)?

What is the best approach to mentor nurses in the science of caring?

How are caring relationships with health care providers best sustained over time?

How do outcomes of care differ between those sites that use caring professional practice models and those who don't?

What research designs best answer caring research questions?

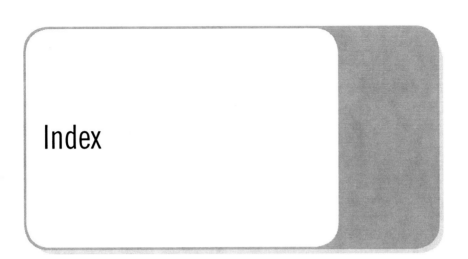

Index